The Language of Medicine

The Language of Medicine

Its Evolution, Structure and
Dynamics

John H. Dirckx, M.D.
*Medical Director, Student
Health Center,
University of Dayton, Dayton, Ohio*

*Medical Department
Harper & Row, Publishers
Hagerstown, Maryland
New York, San Francisco, London*

76 77 78 79 80 81   10 9 8 7 6 5 4 3 2 1

THE LANGUAGE OF MEDICINE: *Its Evolution, Structure and Dynamics.*

Library of Congress Cataloging in Publication Data

Dirckx, John H   1938–
    The language of medicine.

    Bibliography: p. 145
    Includes indexes.
    1. Medicine—Language. 2. English language—
Etymology. I. Title. [DNLM: 1. Nomenclature.
2. Language. W15 D598L]
R123.D57   610'.1'4   75-37500
ISBN 0-06-140689-9

contents

preface

Despite its somewhat pretentious subtitle, this is not a systematic treatise. Any author so imprudent as to attempt an orderly and thorough examination of the whole subject of medical speech and writing would surely exhaust his readers long before exhausting his subject matter. It has been my purpose rather to present a sampling of what is most characteristic and most fascinating about medical language, in as informal and diverting a manner as is consistent with accuracy. Though I have sketched out and generally kept to a logical scheme, I have often deliberately abandoned the well-trodden highway of dictionary and textbook language to wander along the lanes and byways in search of the quaint and the curious, of unusual word origins and quirks of usage.

The language of modern American medicine is an amalgam of words and roots from dozens of ancient and modern languages, a distillate of three thousand years of cultural and linguistic evolution and of almost as long a period of scientific and technical progress. For all that, it is predominantly English, and I have chosen to set the stage for a consideration of medical language with a chapter on the history and chief characteristics of lay, nontechnical or "plain" English. The reader who is interested only in medical terminology may prefer to omit this first chapter.

Similarly, the last chapter may not be particularly appealing to the reader who is impatient of orthographic and grammatical restrictions, who converses by choice in the banal and turbid idiom of the six o'clock news, and whose taste in reading matter runs to Medicare handbooks and advertisements for proprietary headache remedies. At first I had no thought of introducing any critical observations, much less of offering prescriptions for the clear and effective use of language. But as soon as I began gathering material I was struck by the number and variety of faulty or objectionable usages current in medical speech and writing, and when I had put the most flagrant of them together and ventured to suggest how they might be rectified, the result was the longest chapter of all.

Though the nonphysician will, I hope, find here both instruction and entertainment, this book is addressed especially to members of the medical profession. The physician who would ply his art with a steady and tranquil mind, preserving his equanimity in spite of his blunders and failures and never losing sight of the essential worth and dignity even of God's most pusillanimous and exasperating creatures, must become something more than a scientist and a technician: he must be a philosopher and a humanist as well. Of all the manifestations of the grandeur and profundity of the human spirit, none is more ubiquitous, none more revealing than language—the miracle of interpersonal communication through articulate speech, the no less wondrous phenomenon of writing, the staggering diversity of the world's tongues and the timelessness of their literatures.

Thomas Mann wrote that speech is civilization itself. Just as we can learn much about a person's character and attainments by observing carefully how he speaks and writes, so we can gain valuable insight into the mind and soul of a nation, a race, of mankind itself, through the study of language. If we take seriously the old Greek exhortation, "Know thyself," what better language to start with than our own?

The Language of Medicine

1
plain english

History

*The English language, it should be realized, is not
a wayside tree that has grown up wild; it is, rather, a
highly cultivated plant which has been crossbred with
other languages, which has for centuries been grafted and
pruned, and which has been forced in its growth in a soil
fertilized by classical culture. Surely the stages in its
growth and the processes employed in its development de-
serve to be more widely known.*

George H. McKnight
Modern English in the Making (1)

The first mention of what we now call England in the work of a
professional historian occurs in Julius Caesar's COMMENTARIES ON
THE GALLIC WARS. Better known to posterity as a maker of history than
as a writer of it, Caesar himself led Roman troops across the Straits of
Dover in 55 B.C. to begin the military subjection of Britain. Before
turning his attention to this island at the western extremity of the
known world, he had systematically subdued the three parts of Gaul,
which comprised virtually all of continental Europe west of the Rhine
and north of the Pyrenees. The people of Gaul were members of the
Celtic race, and the aboriginal Britons, Caesar's *Britanni,* belonged to
the Cymric branch of the same race, of which the Welsh are the only
surviving representatives.

Around the middle of the first century A.D., during the reign of
the Emperor Claudius, extensive Roman colonies were established in
Britain. In time the native islanders found themselves totally subju-
gated to Roman rule and their territories annexed to the Empire.

1. McKnight GH: MODERN ENGLISH IN THE MAKING. Copyright 1928, renewed
© 1956. Reprinted by permission of Prentice-Hall, Inc., Englewood Cliffs, NJ

Though many of them learned the language of their masters and absorbed some of their culture, the Romanization of Britain was never quite complete. The Picts and Scots, half-savage tribes that inhabited what is now Scotland, retreated into the bleak and desolate highlands where the invaders saw no point in pursuing them.

During the fifth century the Romans, their continental empire tottering on the brink of collapse, abandoned Britain. Although this meant that Rome no longer exacted tribute or imposed its legal system upon the Britons, it also resulted in the withdrawal of the powerful defensive machinery that had kept the Picts and Scots at bay. When these marauding tribes from the north discovered that their forays were no longer opposed by Roman troops, they grew bolder and began to migrate to the south.

The Britons pleaded with Rome to send back a few legions for their protection, but in vain. Their only recourse was to enlist the aid of the hardy, rough-and-tumble seafarers who appeared on their coasts from time to time from across the North Sea. These visitors, natives of northern Germany and Scandinavia, were a Teutonic people very different from both the Celts and the Romans. Large-limbed and blond, perfectly inured to the hardships of the northern climate, they farmed little, rode without saddles, and settled their differences with clubs. Like their cousins the Vikings, they were inveterate wanderers and skillful navigators.

As might have been expected, these formidable Teutonic allies soon became invaders in their own right. The first of them to make trouble were the Jutes, a tribe from the upper Rhine Valley (not from modern Jutland). At the invitation of Vortigern, one of the British kings, an army of Jutes led by Hengist and Horsa had crossed over to England in 449 and successfully beaten back the daring and rapacious Picts and Scots. By way of reward Vortigern had ceded to them the Isle of Thanet, but they soon grew dissatisfied with this small territory and eventually took control of all the land from the Thames estuary south to the Straits of Dover, founding the kingdom of Kent.

In 477 a party of Saxons under the leadership of Aella arrived from northern Germany and established themselves west of Kent. In time their domain came to be called Sussex (southern Saxons); the distinction was necessary because in 495 other Saxons arrived under Cerdic to settle further west (in Wessex), and later invasions by still other Saxons resulted in conquest and colonization of part of the eastern coast of Britain north of the Thames estuary (Essex).

At about the same time, other hordes of Teutons from what is now Schleswig-Holstein were swarming into northern Britain. These people, the Angles, eventually gained control of by far the widest territories, and their three kingdoms, Northumbria, East Anglia and Mercia, extended from the Saxon frontier all the way into Scotland.

The seven kingdoms of the Anglo-Saxon "heptarchy" must not be thought of as political units with fixed borders coexisting in peace and harmony. The various parties of Germanic invaders had much less difficulty in snatching territory from the natives than in keeping it out of each other's hands, and a more or less continual state of war existed for about three centuries.

Eventually the invaders expelled the Britons from all of England except the barren but mineral-rich western districts of Wales and Cornwall. Scholars are not certain what language the Britons spoke when the first of the Germanic invaders arrived—whether they had returned to the Celtic speech of their forefathers or had kept up the Latin of their long-time Roman masters. But it is a matter of historical fact that, with a few trifling exceptions, neither the native Celtic language nor Imperial Latin left any trace on the language spoken throughout most of Britain after the Teutonic invasions.

Surviving Celtic languages are Welsh, spoken today by perhaps a quarter of the people living in Wales; Scots–Gaelic; Irish; Manx, a nearly extinct dialect of the Isle of Man; and Breton, spoken by about a million inhabitants of Brittany on the French coast. (Breton is not a survival of a continental Celtic (Gallic) language, but was carried to France in the fifth and sixth centuries by Welsh and Cornish refugees.) Some words *(e.g., slogan, whisky)* have come into English from these modern Celtic languages in comparatively recent times. Though a few others *(iron, gravel)* seem to have been picked up from the native British Celts by the Teutonic invaders, the total number of such remnants in modern English is extremely small.

Apparently the only traces of Latin left from the Roman occupation of Britain are in place names. For example, *castra = camp* appears in *Winchester, Lancaster, Leicester* and *Exeter,* and *strata via = paved road* in *Stratford* and *street.*

After the sixth century most of the inhabitants of Britain spoke a Teutonic language imported from northern continental Europe. Each of the invading tribes had its own dialect, but all of these dialects shared the same syntactic basis and had many words in common. When, early in the ninth century, the seven Teutonic kingdoms finally resolved their territorial disputes and formed a single nation, they accepted Egbert, who ruled Wessex from 802 to 839, as their first king. (The present royal family of Great Britain can trace its ancestry in an unbroken line back to Egbert.) Though a Saxon kingdom thus achieved political dominance, the Angles occupied by far the greater part of Britain, and it was they who gave their name to the new nation: Angle-land, or England. So also the designation Englisc, or English, was applied to the West Saxon (Wessex) dialect that became the common language of Anglo-Saxon learning and literature and eventually evolved into modern English.

Before we examine some of the characteristics of this Anglo-Saxon language, or Old English, let us view it in perspective. Though the ancient British Celts and their Roman and Germanic invaders had no suspicion of it, all of their languages were related. Modern philology can demonstrate beyond any doubt that these languages had a common parent tongue, which died out long before the dawn of written literature. In fact, the family of languages to which these three belonged, the Aryan (also called Indo-Germanic or Indo-European), embraces nearly every language spoken today in the Western world. Sanskrit, the oldest known representative of the Aryan language family, is the ancestor of modern Hindustani and the other Indic languages. We have already mentioned three other large groups within the family: the Celtic (Welsh, Gaelic, Irish and Breton), the Germanic (German, Dutch, Swedish, Danish, Norwegian, Icelandic and English), and the Latin or Romance (Latin, Italian, Spanish, Portuguese, French, Provençal and Rumanian). Yet this does not nearly exhaust the list, for the Aryan family also includes the Slavic languages (Russian, Bulgarian, Czech and Polish), the Baltic (Lithuanian and Latvian), Armenian, Greek and Albanian.

Not only is the parent language of all these modern tongues lost, but in many cases, neither is there any trace of the intermediate languages and dialects. For example, though all the Teutonic (Germanic) languages display enough similarity to warrant their inclusion in a separate group, we have no written record of any primitive Germanic tongue from which they all developed, and the existence and the characteristics of such a tongue can be established only by inference.

Around the time that the primeval Germanic speech split off from the Aryan mainstream, it underwent two phonetic shifts that would from that time forward characterize all its many offspring. The first of these was a consonant shift, in which initial consonants underwent a softening, so that, for instance, the Aryan initial *p* was muted into *f*. Thus, the primitive root *PED*=*foot* appears in Sanskrit as *pádah,* in Greek as *pous,* and in Latin as *pes;* but the German *Fusz,* like English *foot,* begins with an *f* sound. As another example, initial *k* sound *(kapalam, kephale, caput)* was softened into *h (Haupt, head).*

It must be borne in mind that when we speak of an Aryan parent tongue and a primitive Germanic tongue, we are referring not to written but to spoken languages. All languages are in essence systems of speech; writing is secondary, a means of recording what is, or could be, said. We tend to lose sight of the derivative character of written "speech" because writing and reading play so prominent a role in our use of language, and also because our own system of writing (spelling) displays such vagaries and inconsistencies that its phonetic origin is sometimes obscured. Consider, for example, the silent letters in *doubt, know, yacht;* quirks of pronunciation like *colonel, women;* and the inconsistency of phonetic symbolism exemplified by the series *cough, rough, through, though, bough, bought.*

Of course, visible signs used to communicate ideas need not be phonetic symbols; the Chinese "alphabet" is not phonetic, nor were the runes of the primitive Teutons. Indeed, intelligible signs need have no verbal associations of any sort. Precisely because the black band that distinguishes the oil-immersion objective of a microscope and the green color that identifies an oxygen cylinder are nonverbal symbols, they are universally, or at least internationally, understood.

The second important phonetic change was a shift of stress or accent to the first syllable of a word, which remains today as a distinctive trait of all Germanic languages, including our own. Thus, in compound words like *countryman, daylight,* or *weekend,* we naturally accent the first syllable even though it is obviously not the most important part of the word. Nouns and verbs in Germanic languages that are not customarily accented on the first syllable are almost invariably loan-words from other languages. In fact, many English words derived from non-Teutonic sources have had their accents shifted forward, and many more *(address, adult, detail, research)* are presently undergoing this process, though the practice of accenting these latter words on the first syllable is still widely considered improper.

By the sixth century the Teutonic colonists in Britain had acquired, from Christian missionaries, the art of writing. The very considerable body of literature that has survived from the Anglo-Saxon period enables us to study in detail the primitive tongue from which our modern English is directly descended.

Anglo-Saxon was a highly inflected language. Persons whose knowledge of language is confined to modern English are apt to find the concept of inflection alien and obscure. Inflection is a regular system of changes made in a word to denote changes in its meaning or in its relation to other words in a sentence. Though our language has lost most of its inflections, a few vestiges remain: the *s* that we add to nouns to make them plural; the *'s* by which we signify possession; the *s* that distinguishes the first person singular of a verb in the present tense *(I find, you find, he finds)* and the *–ed* added to a verb to indicate the past tense. We may also mention the irregular plurals *oxen* and *children;* Biblical words like *hast, hath, doth* and *saith;* and changes in pronouns: *he, his, him.*

These are all instances of external flection; that is, they are changes added on to the stem (2) of the word like the endings of the Latin verb that many readers will have learned to conjugate by rote in high school: *amo,* I love; *amas,* you love; *amat,* he loves, etc. Most Anglo-Saxon flections were of this type, though like modern German, the Anglo-Saxon language also had internal flections in which the stem itself underwent a modification, usually a vowel change. We have remnants of this process in modern English in the irregular plurals *mice, geese, men,* and in the past tense of most verbs that do not add *–ed: came, taught, fell.* Though these traces of inflection in modern English are so scanty that it is generally called an uninflected language, Anglo-Saxon, like classical Latin and Greek, and modern German and the Romance languages, employed an extensive inflectional system. It changed nouns and adjectives to denote number (singular or plural), gender (masculine, feminine, or neuter), and case (function in a sentence), while verbs were altered to denote number, person, tense, voice and mood.

A notable trait of Anglo-Saxon was its freedom in forming self-explanatory compounds like our *handbook, horseshoe, shoemaker,* a feature that yet today characterizes the Germanic languages as a class. Anglo-Saxon was extremely rich in synonyms that could be used to express delicate shades of meaning. In BEOWULF, one of the classic verse compositions in Anglo-Saxon, there are thirty-six different words, very few of them compounds or derived forms, for "hero."

Much of the surviving literature in this vigorous and versatile language is poetry. Prose works of note include THE ECCLESIASTICAL HISTORY OF THE ENGLISH PEOPLE written in Latin by the Venerable Bede around 730 and early translated into "English," and the ANGLO-SAXON CHRONICLE, prepared under the direction of King Alfred (who reigned 871–901). From these two records much of the historical material in this chapter is ultimately derived.

2. Though *stem* and *root* are often used interchangeably, they have specific and different meanings in linguistics. A stem is what is left of a word after all inflectional endings have been removed; a root is a basic phonetic component of two or more words that are related in origin and meaning. The root *CALC* appears in both *calcium* and *calculus.* Often a root has a labile vowel: *HID/HYD* as in *hydrogen, hydatid, hidradenitis.*

Here is a brief passage from the close of the latter work, which relates the death of Alfred:

> 901. Her gefor Aelfred Athulfing, syx nihtum aer ealra haligra maessan. Se waes cyning ofer eall Ongelcyn butan thaem daele the under Dena onwalde waes, ond he heold thaet rice othrum healfum laes the .xxx. wintra. Ond tha feng Eadweard, his sunu, to rice.
>
> (901. Here [*i.e.,* in this year] died Alfred, son of Athelwulf, six nights before the feast of All Saints. He was king over all the English nation except the part that was in the power of the Danes, and he reigned a year and a half less than thirty years. And then began Edward, his son, to reign.)

This specimen of Anglo-Saxon is presented to show how much it differs from our own language, even though modern English is descended directly from it. Only four words *(under, he, his, to)* have come down to us with spelling unchanged. (Anglo-Saxon *the* is not our definite article but an obsolete form of our words *than* and *that.*) Some do not differ greatly from their modern counterparts *(her, waes, ofer, ond, sunu),* while others are barely recognizable *(cyning=king; healfum= half).* And though there is scarcely a word here that has not a descendant in modern English, our general impression is that we are looking at a "foreign" language. Indeed, almost any book in modern Danish or Dutch will contain passages that are more readily intelligible to the English-speaking reader than this sample of Old English.

Languages, like wines, grow easier on the tongue with age. The mellowing process does not, of course, proceed according to fixed rules; but with due allowance for the effects of ethnic, geographic, and political influences, it is generally true to say that the evolution and differentiation of any language involves most or all of the following processes: changes in the meaning of words, especially by metaphoric extension; borrowing of new words and roots from other languages; coinage of new words, derivatives, and compounds; loss of inflections and relaxation of grammatical "rules". All of these processes were operative in the evolution of Middle English from Old English, as we are about to see.

Although the syntactic structure of a living language at any given time always represents a simplification of some previous system, the fact may not be obvious if the previous system has been entirely lost. To complicate the matter further, languages become simpler by two alternate processes, the one synthetic and the other analytic, which seem the very reverse of each other. For example, in Aryan languages virtually all inflectional endings are actually included words or word fragments. In the conjugation of the Latin verb, the endings are thought to represent primitive pronouns that came to be so closely associated with the verb stem that they fused with it: *am+ego=amo.* This is a synthetic process and in its way it represents a simplification, since it says with one word what formerly required two. In conjugating a Greek verb it is necessary to add to the stem a variety of reduplications, augments, thematic vowels, tense signs and personal endings. Though some of these elements are purely phonetic expedients, many of them must be rudimentary words like our auxiliary verbs *have, had, been, will,* etc.

The terminations of Latin nouns—the "case endings"—are probably absorbed prepositions. The height of elegance in classical Latin was to omit prepositions almost entirely, and to signify relationships between nouns by adroit use of the oblique cases. Many modern languages, including English, do somewhat the same: "Give [to] me the book"; "Let's make [for] him a prosthesis." Classical Latin had no word for *of* in the possessive sense, as in "the wealth of George." (Again, English usually expresses this relation with the possessive case-ending *'s:* "George's wealth.") But the highly polished and artificial Latin of the Augustan Age was descended from a much earlier language, a purely spoken idiom in which many prepositions must have existed that eventually came to be absorbed into the ends of nouns to express different meanings, and so yielded the changes in nouns that we call declension. So much for simplification by synthesis.

When the original sense of the absorbed words and word fragments is obscured by the passage of time, inflection comes to be a hindrance rather than a help to simpler expression, because it seems to be an arbitrary system in which form and meaning are unrelated. Then begins the analytic process. The inflectional forms, their utility lost with their significance, are chopped down to stem words again, and the prepositions and pronouns in current use are employed to indicate relationships among them. It was this analytic process, operative from about the tenth to the fifteenth century, that was responsible for the loss of Anglo-Saxon inflections. In the languages descended from Latin the process has nearly abolished the inflection of nouns, though with the exception of spoken French the modern Romance languages still maintain a fairly complete system of verb inflection.

The reader will have noted in the extract from the ANGLO-SAXON CHRONICLE that the domain of King Alfred did not include the part of Britain under Danish rule. About 787, even before the consolidation of the English nation under Egbert, another band of Teutonic invaders, the Danes, appeared on British shores. As they found most of the country already occupied by the Anglo-Saxons, they established only a few independent settlements in what is now Lincolnshire. Nevertheless through gradual infiltration and domination they eventually took over the whole country. Though in Alfred's time the Danish territory, or Danelaw, comprised only the northeast portion of England, by the end of the tenth century the Danes had brought the entire nation under their control, and between 1016 and 1042 three Danish kings in succession sat on the English throne.

But the Danes made no attempt to drive out the Anglo-Saxons, who came of the same racial stock as themselves. The language of these new invaders was very similar to Anglo-Saxon, but because there was already a substantial literature in Anglo-Saxon we can judge which Teutonic words came into English at the time of the Danish invasion and which were there before it. The consensus of scholars is that Danish did not contribute a great many words, though it did give us a few of our most common ones *(die, hit, ill, low, take, window)*. The Danes also introduced a few variant forms which appear in some of the interesting cognate doublets that so abound in English: from Anglo-Saxon, *whole, no, shirt, shriek;* from Danish, *hale, nay, skirt, screech.* A number of words in the Scots dialect *(e.g., bairn=child* and *maun=must)* are of Danish origin.

It was only twenty-four years after the Anglo-Saxons had regained control of the throne of England under Edward the Confessor that an event occurred which was to exert a much more profound influence upon the language of England than the Danish occupation. In 1066 William the Conqueror invaded England at the head of an army of Normans and achieved a complete victory, mounting the English throne as William I.

These Normans were a roving, adventurous people from the coast of France, but they were not of French stock. Late in the ninth century a band of Scandinavian wanderers led by Rollo had drifted into northwestern France. By 912 these Northmen, or Normans, had so completely taken possession of the region around the Seine estuary that King Charles the Simple ceded the territory to them, and it is known as Normandy to this day. Never content to stay at home and lead the simple life, the Normans went on in their old ways; at about the same time that William was winning the Battle of Hastings, another Norman, Robert Guiscard, was subduing southern Italy.

The outcome of the Norman Conquest was in sharp contrast to that of the Teutonic invasions of five centuries earlier. Whereas the

Angles and Saxons had practically exterminated the Celtic Britons, herding the survivors into the northern and western wilds, the Normans were content merely to enslave the English. Although the Normans were of Teutonic origin like their new vassals, the language they spoke was a dialect of French which soon came to be the language of learning and culture in England, and continued so, with a strong influence on the Anglo-Saxon still spoken by the unlettered majority, until the fourteenth century.

Let us take a look at this Norman French which was to exert so powerful an influence upon our own language. During the centuries since Julius Caesar had first carried the Latin of Imperial Rome on to British soil, that language had undergone a remarkable series of changes. Once a fairly uniform idiom throughout the vast Roman Empire (3), it had gradually acquired regional peculiarities and broken up into numerous dialects. As time went on some of these dialects fused, others drifted further apart, and still others died out. By the end of the Dark Ages, Latin no longer existed as a spoken language; in its place remained five distinct languages, each bound to a geopolitical or ethnic group: Italian, Spanish, Portuguese, French, and Rumanian.

Between the third and fifth centuries the Romanization of Gaul gradually extinguished all traces of the primitive Celtic language of the inhabitants. Though the oldest specimen of written French is the Oath of Strasbourg (842), the French language already existed in the fifth century as a "Gallic" dialect of Late Latin. By 500 A.D. the Latin of Gaul had not only evolved into primitive French, but displayed two rather distinct dialectal variants. The northern one was characterized by a shift from the *a* of Latin to *e* or *ie:* Latin *mare=sea* and *canis=dog* became *mer* and *chien.* In the southern dialect, spoken by people closer to the Italian peninsula, this shift had not taken place. The two dialects were and are distinguished by their respective words for *yes,* the southern being known as Languedoc (the language of *oc*) and the northern as Languedoil (the language of *oil,* modern *oui*). Languedoc formed the basis of Provençal, the language of the medieval troubadours, which survives as a group of dialects still spoken in southern France.

It was during the fourth century that the Franks, who eventually gave their name to France, appeared on the banks of the Rhine. Like

3. The language spoken throughout the western half of the Roman Empire during the first and second centuries A.D. was not the Latin of Cicero and Virgil, but a vernacular which philologists (from their exalted position) now call Low Latin. It is doubtful that the highly refined but stilted language of literature and oratory cultivated during the Augustan Age was ever a medium of informal daily conversation.

the Angles and the Saxons, the Danes and the Normans, these were yet another Teutonic people. Ostensibly allies of the Romans, or at least mercenaries in the service of Caesar, they were chiefly interested in plunder and in extending their frontiers into more temperate latitudes.

It is not mere coincidence that in tracing the history of our language we so often encounter migrating tribes of Teutons. The great southwest migration of the Germanic tribes was one of the most historic events of the Christian era, ranking with the establishment of Islam and the discovery of America. We must not think of these half-savage northerners as riding at full gallop with drawn swords across three thousand miles of Europe, spreading slaughter and destruction everywhere. Their swarming across the European continent and their eventual conquest of much of it was a gradual process, a sort of chain reaction touched off when the Huns, a fierce, nomadic race of north central Asia, migrated into the Volga valley late in the fourth century. The tribes displaced by the Huns moved south and west to displace other tribes in their turn. Besides precipitating the migration of the Franks into Gaul, the Huns drove the Visigoths into Spain, the Ostrogoths into Italy and Hungary, and the Vandals as far as North Africa. The Germanic invasions were the most decisive factor in the collapse of the Roman Empire, and there is not a language, a culture, or a nation in modern Europe that has not been deeply influenced by them.

First united under Clovis in 481, the Franks proceeded to conquer most of west central Europe, including what is now France and Germany. Though they imposed their rule upon the people of Gaul, they did not impose their language. The developing French tongue borrowed a number of Frankish words, but modern French is still predominantly a Romance (Latin) language. The French words *garçon, guerre* and *hangar,* whose meanings are familiar to most speakers of English, are from Frankish, not Latin, roots.

By the tenth century the number of French dialects had risen to four: Parisian or Île-de-France, Picard, Burgundian and Norman. Around the thirteenth century it appeared that Norman would eventually win out and become the common speech of all France, but modern French is actually a descendant of the Île-de-France dialect.

It was Norman, of course, and not Parisian French that served as the "official" language of England during the eleventh and twelfth centuries. Though the House of Normandy retained possession of the English throne for less than a hundred years, ceding to the Plantagenets in 1154, the first Plantagenet king, Henry II, inherited control of much of France. Even after Henry's son and successor John, by one of the diplomatic blunders that earned him the epithet "Lackland," lost control of Normandy and the other French possessions of the English crown early in the thirteenth century, Norman continued to be spoken in England by the wealthy and the literate. Indeed, it survived as the language of law until the sixteenth century, and many modern legal terms are relics of "Law French": *arraign, escheat, malfeasance, mortgage, tort.*

But the Anglo-Saxon language had never died out. It had continued to be the medium of daily speech among the common people, and it began to flourish again as a written language in the fourteenth century, when the first great writers of English—Langland, Gower, Chaucer and Mandeville—used it as a literary vehicle. Though Anglo-Saxon had survived the long Norman interlude, it had not come unchanged through the centuries. In fact, when we rediscover it in the works of these fourteenth century authors, it has undergone a remarkable metamorphosis: it has absorbed thousands of Romance words and roots from French, lost most of its inflectional system, and evolved so far in the direction of our own modern English that we can now make shift to read it without much difficulty. So great a change of structure warrants a change of name as well; the English of the fourteenth century is called Middle English to distinguish it from Anglo-Saxon or Old English and from modern English.

The following passage is taken from the Prologue to Chaucer's great work, THE CANTERBURY TALES. Except for the use of modern letters in place of the old symbols for *gh* and *th,* the passage appears exactly as it was written in 1387, more than a century before Columbus discovered America. Besides displaying very well the character of Middle English, it is an excellent specimen of Chaucer's droll wit.

> With us ther was a Doctour of Physik:
> In all this world ne was ther noon hym lik (4),
> To speke of physik and of surgerye;
> For he was grounded in astronomye . . .
> He knew the cause of everich maladye,
> Were it of hoot, or cold, or moyste, or drye,
> And where they engendred and of what
>   humour;
> He was a verray parfit praktisour . . .
> Of his diete mesurable was he,
> For it was of no superfluitee,

---

4. *I.e.,* "there was none like him." The double negative *(ne . . .noon)* was common in Middle English. Those who know some French may suspect that this usage was due to the Norman influence, but in fact it was common in Anglo-Saxon also.

But of great norissyng and digestible.
His studie was but litel on the Bible.

The history of the English language after the time of Chaucer is essentially the history of England itself and of its rich and varied literature. By the end of the fourteenth century, the language had already received its distinctive character as a blend of two disparate linguistic strains, the Teutonic and the Romance, in an incredibly happy marriage destined to be blessed with many offspring in the languages and dialects of England, Scotland, Ireland, Australia, Canada and the United States. To pursue its history further in a chronologic fashion would carry us far afield, and we now shift our frame of reference to examine the form and function of modern English.

𝔓𝔥𝔶𝔰𝔦𝔠𝔞𝔩 𝔈𝔵𝔞𝔪𝔦𝔫𝔞𝔱𝔦𝔬𝔫

The English language is a methodical, energetic, business-like and sober language, that does not care much for finery and elegance, but does care for logical consistency and is opposed to any attempt to narrow-in life by police regulations and strict rules either of grammar or of lexicon.

Otto Jespersen
Growth and Structure of the English Language (5)

We native speakers of English are an arrogant crowd. We expect visitors from other countries to understand and speak our language, but we cannot be troubled to learn theirs when we go abroad. We ridicule foreigners who stumble over our erratic "rules" of pronunciation and mangle our many complicated idioms. Indeed, dozens of comedians and professional dialecticians make their livings by mimicking the errors characteristically made by Italians, Germans, Japanese and Swedes struggling with the phonetics of English.

Whereas the Dutch, the Swiss and the Scandinavians are forced by sheer practical necessity to become reasonably proficient in three or more languages, Americans have no such incentives. The teaching of foreign languages in this country is often conducted in a half-hearted and thoroughly incompetent fashion, and educators themselves proba-

5. Jespersen O: GROWTH AND STRUCTURE OF THE ENGLISH LANGUAGE, 9th ed. Riverside, NJ, © The Free Press, Macmillan, 1968

bly do not believe in some of the motivations they try to foist on students for acquiring fluency in a foreign language. No American needs to speak another language when he travels, for English is spoken in every country of the world. No American with less than a professional interest in a foreign literature needs to learn the language in which it is written, because practically everything worth reading is available in English translation. Nor is a young person without special linguistic aptitudes and interests likely to pursue language study for career advancement.

It goes without saying that the losses resulting from our linguistic parochialism are all our own. Our cultural horizons are narrowly limited by our reluctance to get into the mental and linguistic skin of another race or nation. Our capacity for understanding the cultural heritages, the ethnic traits and the national aspirations of other peoples is severely hampered by our inability to "think in their language." It was a king who said, "To possess another language is to possess another soul."

Moreover, unilingualism renders one incapable of seeing even his own language in its true colors. Perhaps no tongue ever spoken on earth was so rich, so plastic, so expressive as English. But for a person who knows no other language than English, its unique beauties and strengths must remain largely unappreciated. Furthermore, its faults as a medium of expression (and it has them in plenty) are readily overlooked by persons desirous of improving their speaking and writing skills if they confine their attention to English syntax alone.

Let us count over some of the features that make English the remarkably variegated, beautiful and serviceable language that it is. There is such an abundance of these features that I have been obliged to pick and choose those that seem most characteristic to me. This is rather like trying to paint a portrait by showing one ear, one eye and the tip of the nose. Inevitably, the selection reflects the tastes and also betrays the prejudice and ignorance of the chooser.

Most of the truly conspicuous and unique characteristics of our language arise from one single circumstance: that it is a hybrid tongue composed of the best and worst of two widely differing linguistic strains, the Teutonic and the Romance. The traditional contrast between the fair, taciturn, stubborn, saturnine, warlike Teuton and the dark, voluble, mercurial, genial, passionate Latin is a little overworked, but like most clichés it contains a generous share of truth.

The Germanic invaders of Britain were a shrewd and practical people who probably looked upon their system of speech as no more intellectual or spiritual an entity than an axe or an oar. Though the language they brought with them was a highly articulate one with a complex inflectional system and a rich lexicon, it had undergone important phonetic changes since splitting off from the Aryan parent language. Some of these have already been mentioned. It was formerly believed that primitive Germanic was largely composed of monosyllables, but this view was based upon insufficient evidence. It now appears that the primitive speech of the northern barbarians was rich in polysyllabic words, and did not break up into shorter fragments until after these tribes had come into contact with more civilized peoples. Be that as it may, Anglo-Saxon was rugged, harsh, monosyllabic and guttural.

By contrast, the Romance languages were born and bred in the countries of the Mediterranean littoral, whose climate and other physical features allowed the inhabitants leisure to cultivate conversation as an art form, and to develop a literature rich in epic, lyrical and elegiac poetry and drama at a time when Teutonic "literature" was limited to the rude effusions of hunters and warriors gathered at the tribal fireside. Primeval Latin, like Greek, was fluid, melodious and polysyllabic.

The contrast between English words of Teutonic origin and those of Romance origin can be seen in the following pairs of synonyms: *house–domicile, show–demonstrate, trust–confidence, fair–equitable.* Though this demonstration illustrates the point strikingly enough, it is a little contrived, and proves nothing. So completely have the two elements mingled in modern English, and so far has the language evolved and matured, that with a little effort one might select a list of synonym pairs that seemed to prove the opposite thesis.

Romance (predominantly French) elements have been so completely assimilated into the basic language that only a philologist can distinguish them from native (Germanic) stock. Some words taken from medieval Norman are spelled in English exactly as are their descendants in modern French: *age, air, large, place, point.* Others have been recast in the Anglo-Saxon mold, so that even a Frenchman cannot recognize them: *abridge, budge, curfew, haughty, powder, wig.* English has freely formed compounds between French words and native Anglo-Saxon affixes, as in *beautiful, courtly,* and *napkin.* Contrariwise, many Latin and French particles are living affixes in English, and have been applied to words and roots of Anglo-Saxon origin: *defrost, starvation* and *unbreakable.*

Words of purely Teutonic descent tend to be more vigorous, masculine and explicit than Romance words. In fact, though about half the words in the English dictionary may be of Romance origin, most of the ones we use in everyday speech are Teutonic. Nearly all English pronouns, prepositions and conjunctions are from Teutonic stock, as are a substantial majority of nouns, verbs and adjectives referring to common things. When we shout in anger or groan in pain, we use an almost purely Anglo-Saxon speech.

Even before the accession of words borrowed or coined from classic Latin to meet the requirements of advancing science and technology, words derived from Romance roots had seemed better fit for the expression of abstract or complex ideas in the physical sciences, philosophy and art. Nowadays they are also the usual medium of sophisticated (and snobbish and pompous) speech and writing. Euphemisms are quite generally Romance words, which often seem more genteel, or at least less blunt, than their Germanic counterparts. (Most physicians would rather ask a patient whether he has a family history of *seizures* than inquire about *fits,* and most would rather discuss a *malodor* than a *stink.*) Premeditated insolence, satire and the mock-heroic all make heavy use of Romance words.

English is unique among Germanic languages in not forming most of its compound words out of native Teutonic stock. The noun corresponding to *go down* is *descent* (or *decline*); we have no synonym built up from Anglo-Saxon material. Similarly, our noun for *go away* is *departure* (or *recession*) and for *go in, entry.* In each of these cases, the only way to express with a noun the action denoted by the verb is to use either a Romance word or a gerund (*going down,* etc.).

Other Germanic languages build up compound words from native stock for many concepts that we can hardly express at all without recourse to Romance compounds: compare German *Erziehung,* English *education; wiederholen, repeat; verschieden, different; ausschlieszlich, exclusively.* Not only does English prefer Romance forms to native compounds in these cases, but even for simple Anglo-Saxon verbs in everyday use English customarily fabricates the corresponding nouns and adjectives from Romance material: *get–reception; see–visible; can–possible; have–possessive; be–nonexistence.* This is one of the chief reasons why a speaker of English experiences much less difficulty in acquiring a working vocabulary in a Romance language than in learning the same number and kind of words in German.

With its extremely rich heritage of words and roots, English has more different ways of saying things than most languages. This makes it a more difficult language to learn well, because each variant mode of expression has its connotation established by convention, and unless one knows the nuances of meaning attached to these different forms, he cannot make effective use of them. But this wealth of synonyms allows a native speaker of English to express himself both more succinctly and more precisely.

The translation of a novel from English to Spanish fills ten or fifteen percent more pages than the original. The reason is that Spanish, though a language of great power and beauty, has comparatively little flexibility of expression, and is obliged to employ many tiresome circumlocutions to say what can be compressed easily into a word or two in English. A speaker of Spanish may contrive to lop off a syllable here and a word there, but written Spanish is expected to conform to the Grammar and Dictionary of the Royal Spanish Academy. Because the Academy will accept only words and usages of great venerability and untarnished pedigree, its dictionary, supposedly comprising the entire Spanish language, is only a fraction of the size of THE OXFORD ENGLISH DICTIONARY, partly because English, by contrast, has always been broadly tolerant of variant forms, coinages, and downright slang.

The diversity of origin of our words makes for a diversity of sounds. Not only is the relation between English spelling and pronunciation extremely erratic, but English has a much broader range of acceptable or "correct" pronunciations. Does your son have a paper *root* or *rowt?* Does your wife want a new dining-room *soot* or *sweet?* Compare pronunciations listed in various dictionaries for *envelope, gaseous, harass, lamentable, nausea.*

A novelist who wishes to create a stark and grim atmosphere uses Anglo-Saxon words like *stark* and *grim,* but if he wants to convey an impression of languorous ease or pensive tranquillity he resorts to Romance words. A poet in need of an extra syllable can generally find a suitable alternative word that contains it. Indeed, English poetry displays a much wider diversity of rhythms and rhyme schemes than that of any other language. German, French and Italian each have their characteristic cadences, and the poetry of each is ineluctably bound to its phonetic heritage.

By no means all of the features peculiar to English are due to the mingling of Teutonic and Romance lexical material. A widow is *bereaved;* a maniac is *bereft* of his senses. We say *"burnt* toast" but "a *burned* child." A person may be *struck* by a car or *stricken* with cancer. These passive participle pairs are not merely variant spellings like *gray* and *grey.* They are two lexical forms of the same word with slightly different meanings established by long usage, and it is just this delicate hue and shade of distinction in meaning between words of identical origin that imparts to English much of its incomparable expressiveness and plasticity.

But though the person whose mother tongue is English may well rejoice in these precious linguistic resources, the foreign medical graduate struggling to master the vagaries of English vocabulary will probably entertain less enthusiastic views. These vagaries can be confusing at times even for native speakers of English, as witness the following excerpt from a physical examination report: "Several small, firm, discreet, non-tender nodes are palpable in the left axilla." *Discreet* and *discrete* are not only members of the same clan as *bereaved–bereft,* but they also have the interesting peculiarity of being pronounced alike. *Discrete* (which yields the derivatives *discreteness* and *non-discrete*) means "distinct" or "separate." *Discreet* (forming *discretion* and *indiscreet*) is defined as "wisely cautious in speech and action." Clearly, the patient's axillary nodes can no more be *discreet* than his skin can be *pail* or his voice *horse* or his knees *week.*

If an athlete catches a ball with his finger *crooked* (one syllable) he may end up with a *crooked* (two syllables) finger. When a family has been *blessed* with a new child, the birth is called a *blesséd* event. In either case, to confound the one-syllable with the two-syllable form would be an error not of spelling but of pronunciation. Finally, if we say a picture was *hanged* on the wall, or that a murderer was *hung,* we may be accused of bad grammar. Yet in all these instances—misspelling, mispronunciation, faulty grammar—the substance of the error is confusion between two passive participle doublets.

The study of these and other kinds of doublets can shed much light on the development and structure of modern English. *Discrete* and *discreet* are homophones; *blessed* and *blesséd* are homographs. Not all homographs are of identical origin, as is illustrated by *periodic = occurring at intervals* and *periodic = iodine-containing radical.*

English has far more true homonyms (sets of words identical in both spelling and pronunciation but different in both origin and meaning) than most other languages; in Chinese, for example, they are impossible. What is chiefly striking about the abundance of homonyms in English is not that they exist but that they cause so little confusion; that the mind is capable of fastening on to clues that enable it automatically to assign the correct one of two or more alternate meanings to a word or sound.

Another source of doublet formation is the borrowing from two different languages of words formed from the same root. We have already mentioned Danish and Anglo-Saxon pairs like *hale–whole.* Another type is seen in *guard–ward* and *guarantee–warranty.* These are words formed from Teutonic roots starting with *w.* Since the initial *w* sound in Frankish words was foreign and practically unpronounceable for the primitive Gauls, they changed it to *gu,* and the *gu* forms like *guard* have come into English by way of French. (Modern French has in many instances dropped the *u;* cf. *avant-garde.*). The corresponding *w* forms entered modern English directly from Anglo-Saxon.

English is extremely rich in idiomatic expressions that employ simple words with specialized meanings. I can take a fancy to a horse, I can take a bale of hay to a horse, or I can take a whip to a horse. You and I may fall into the same error, the same category, or the same ditch. I can give you a black box, a black look, a black mark, or a black eye. You may then go off in a huff, in a while, in a hurry, or in a Jeep. You may be fresh out of school, fresh out of pique, or fresh out of razor blades.

Though all languages have idioms like these, they are especially abundant in English where a great many of them are accepted as part of the polite language. This does not mean that English has proportionately less slang, so recognized, than other languages; in fact it has more slang than any other. The English language is so rich in metaphorical and figurative usages that the speaker and writer must exercise considerable care to avoid mixing them in ludicrous fashion. Preposterous expressions like "Keep *sharp tabs* on him," "We have to *iron out* the *bugs,*" and "He's tired of *playing second fiddle* to *visiting firemen*" are so common that they are intelligible to all but foreigners, who alone perceive their absurdity.

English has a nearly unique ability to diversify the function of a word without changing its form. Since we have dispensed almost entirely with inflections, we must rely on clues derived from word order to decide what function is served by *down* in each of the following expressions: "It's fourth down, fans!" (noun); "I'll down him with one blow," (verb); "Take the down escalator," (adjective); "Jack fell down," (adverb), "Pour it down the drain," (preposition); "Down, Rover!" (interjection).

Other languages, of course, can and do form various parts of speech from the same stem, but generally by making appropriate changes in its form. Though with few exceptions the spelling of an English word gives the reader no hint as to its role in a sentence, there is a large group of words whose function is indicated in speech by the placement of the accent. If we stress the first syllable of *conduct,* we have a noun meaning *behavior;* if we stress the second syllable, we have a verb meaning *lead* or *transport.* In virtually all words in this category, most of them compounds derived from Latin, the rule is that the noun form carries the accent on the first syllable, the verb and adjective forms on the second.

In modern usage there is a strong tendency for this distinction to be lost, as the Germanic penchant for accenting the first syllable of every word spreads by analogy even to words of non-Germanic origin. Thus, we hear of COMplex molecules and COMpact automobiles, of activists who PROtest and uteri that PROlapse, of doctors who ILlustrate articles and of articles that INfluence doctors. If most of these pronunciations grate on refined ears, a few are not without their humorous aspect: a "CONcrete epidemiologic model" is not an epidemiologic model that is *real* but one that is *made of concrete.*

The tendency to eliminate the phonetic distinctions in words of this class has been particularly active in the case of those beginning with *pro–* and *com– (con–)*. Among this group, almost the only words consistently pronounced in accordance with the rule are those that never function as nouns *(complete, protect)* and those whose noun forms are used far less frequently than the verb forms *(convert, proceed)*.

As might be expected, the efforts of purists to reverse this trend in spoken English have proven fruitless. The purists themselves sometimes overdo things a little: an EXpert witness (usual modern pronunciation, incidentally correct) is an expert who serves as a witness; an exPERT witness (pedant's pronunciation) is an expert at being a witness. (In this litigious age, both pronunciations may sometimes be correct.)

Besides making a single form like *down* serve as a word-of-all-work, now using it as a verb, now as an adjective or an adverb, English assigns to many words an extremely broad range of connotations even within the formal boundaries of a single part of speech. The fundamental, transitive meaning of the verb *deliver* is seen in "The clerk delivered the records to the chart desk." By contrast, "We deliver" is an absolute use of the verb, in which an object is understood but not expressed. As an outgrowth of this usage, we have the apparently reflexive sense of the verb seen in "Mrs. Baynes delivered at 4:15." That this is not another example of the merely absolute use, in which "a baby" is understood but not mentioned, seems clear from the fact that in still another variation we can say "Dr. Smith delivered Mrs. Baynes" instead of "Dr. Smith delivered the baby," which latter is not, however, yet a fifth mode of delivering, but the first one over again with a specific obstetric meaning.

A similar set of variations occurs in the following anecdote. "While he was *washing* [himself] he noticed a stain of oil on his sleeve. His wife *washed* [the clothes] next morning, and though she *washed* the shirt carefully, the stain didn't *wash* out." The last use of *wash* illustrates a syntactic figure peculiar to English, in which a fictitious active construction is employed to express a passive idea (the stain *washes*, the tablet *crushes up* easily) or sometimes an instrumental one (the pen *writes*).

Closely akin to these variations on the active–passive theme are words like *shrug* and *wink,* in which the object *(shoulders, eye),* a part of the doer's body, is suppressed. Classic Greek had a middle voice ("between" active and passive) to handle such situations, but in most modern European languages the speaker is obliged to name the direct objects of these verbs, even though nobody could possibly shrug anything but his own shoulders, or wink anything but his own eye.

In the case of *wink* this can be explained by the relative conservatism and explicitness of these languages, as contrasted with English, but *shrug* is a different matter. The reason why it is impossible to translate *shrug* into most modern languages without supplying the object *shoulders* is that these languages express the action of shrugging by a verb with a much wider range of meanings than our verb. The German *jerks* his shoulders, the Frenchman *lifts* his, while the Spaniard, the Italian, the Russian and the Hungarian *contract* theirs. English, notoriously prodigal of its phonetic resources, reserves a special verb for this one application.

To set forth the structure and function of English in this piecemeal fashion may give the illusion that a language is a mere assemblage of words instead of a dynamic and constantly evolving organism, a phenomenon rather than a process. Philologists of the old school cherish that illusion; the Italian, French and Spanish Academies are dedicated to its perpetuation. But the genius of English is not to be hedged in by schoolmarms or trammeled by academicians. This is nowhere more evident than in the rate at which the language grows in sheer bulk.

From the earliest times English has displayed a proclivity for borrowing words from other tongues. Britannia, Mistress of the Waves, either warred or traded with every other nation on earth, and greedily absorbed words from them all, often recasting them in its own mold. Thus the Spanish *cucaracha* becomes *cockroach,* French *écrevisse* turns into *crayfish,* and the Arabic chess expression *shah mat* ("The King is dead") appears in English as *checkmate.*

Other languages were, of course, doing the same thing with English words even before English became an international medium of communication. In German we find *fesch = fashionable,* in Spanish and Portuguese *líder = leader* and in French *bouledogue = bulldog.* The English words *club(= association), jockey, football(=* what Americans call *soccer), interview, revolver* and *whisky* appear in most modern European languages in one form or another. *Redingote,* imported from France several seasons ago as the name of a style of ladies' evening wear, was simply the English *riding coat* as retailored in the eighteenth century for the French tongue and ear. French *biftek* = *beefsteak* and *rosbif* = *roast beef* both contain corruptions of our word *beef,* which is itself a corruption of Norman *boef.*

We have seen already that English has no hesitation about mixing up roots of diverse origins in a single word. Linguistically irregular compounds like *chortle, electrocute, happenstance, paratrooper* and *telethon,* in which word fragments have been slapped together with blithe disregard for their semantic or lexical associations, abound in modern English. Moreover, the language readily tolerates the invention of words like *blurb, zipper* and *quiz* out of thin air.

Like its forebear Anglo-Saxon, English is full of compound expressions and epithets like *butterfingers, numbskull* and *to pussyfoot.* English prefers brief, vigorous modes of speech ("What I say goes"; "Get with it!") to the prolixity and circumlocution favored by some languages, and likes to shorten words to give them more force and poignancy: [*omni*]*bus, champ*[*ion*], *fan*[*atic*], [*chrysanthe*]*mum, pant*[*aloon*]*s,* [*tele*]*phone,* [*cara*]*van, van*[*guard*]. English is one of the few languages whose diminutives are actually smaller in size than the forms from which they are derived. We cut down Elizabeth, Peter and Josephine to *Liz, Pete* and *Jo;* in most languages the diminutive or nickname form is made by adding one or more syllables, like *–chen, –ette,* or *–ino.*

Whole families of English words may grow out of single root words in consequence of the mixing and battering that are inevitable in a language so far-flung geographically and of such various phonetic and ethnic origins. Consider the progeny of the Latin *gentilis* = *belonging to a clan;* later, = *high-minded, noble.* Long before the Norman Conquest, Anglo-Saxon had absorbed the ethnic designation *Gentile* from Bible Latin. When the Normans came they brought their version of the Latin word, *gentil,* and in due course this became a part of Middle English; the modern spelling *(gentle)* appeared in the sixteenth century, and the modern meaning became current at about the same time. Later the French word crossed the Channel yet again, this time retaining its foreign character and also some of its native pronunciation, *zhahn-TEEY.* Phonetic spelling of this French word then gave birth to not one but two new English words, *genteel* and *jaunty.* Meanwhile, *gentility* preserves the original meaning of the stem *(noble birth),* while *gentleness* conveys the more modern sense of *mildness* or *restraint,* and *gentleman* includes both connotations.

2

medical english

Having reviewed the history of modern English and considered some of its distinguishing features, we are now going to see what happens when the English language and the science of medicine come into contact. Our purpose here is to investigate the role of native English words in the technical language of medicine, and to examine the dynamics of English as a medium of technical communication. At the risk of imparting to this chapter the repellent aspect of a textbook, I am going to discuss medical English under the threefold division of nouns, adjectives and verbs.

Nouns

"What's in a name?"

William Shakespeare
Romeo and Juliet

It is self-evident that no matter how thickly we intersperse our speech and writing with technical terms, the underlying foundation or substrate is "plain" English. Moreover, a great many of the technical terms used by speakers of English are words native to the language rather than importations or coinages from the learned tongues. As technical terminology consists principally of nouns, our first and chief concern will be with them.

Many of the terms employed in gross anatomy are words taken from the English common speech: *arm, back, breast, ear, hair, hand, head, neck, rib, scalp, skin, skull, tongue* (1). Physicians almost never call these structures by any other names. For some parts of the body there are no

---

1. Unlike the other words in this list, which are of Anglo-Saxon origin, *scalp, skin* and *skull* are part of our small but valuable legacy from the Danes. Despite its appearance, *tongue* is not French. The *u* was inserted in the Anglo-Saxon word *tonge* around Shakespeare's time, apparently to prevent its being pronounced with a soft *g*.

"polite" English words, so that the anatomist and the physician use either a Latin term *(anus)* or an English word adapted from Latin *(testicle)*. Some English anatomic terms, though perfectly acceptable in polite speech, are by convention applied only to animals. Thus, the physician speaks of his patient's *pancreas,* not his *sweetbreads;* of his *esophagus* rather than his *gullet;* of *cartilage* instead of *gristle.* Though *flank* is also usually reserved by laymen for references to animals, the medical profession uses it as a human anatomic designation: *flank pain* is a common enough expression in the language of medicine, yet it is likely to be unintelligible to many laymen.

Most internal organs and tissues have native English designations also: *gallbladder, liver, spleen; blood, bone, fat.* The anatomist is obliged to use non-English terms for only two kinds of structure: those whose existence was not generally known to laymen during the formative period of the language, and those for which the available native English word is not sufficiently specific. *Adrenal, ovary* and *prostate* are in the first category, as are all the structures revealed by the microscope.

To the second category belong such terms as *duodenum, jejunum, ileum* and *colon* (which convey more specific information than the general word *bowel*), and *tendon,* which is only one of the structures called *sinews* by the Anglo-Saxons, the others being *ligaments* and *nerves.* (Etymologically, *nerve* is no more appropriate a designation than Anglo-Saxon *sionu. Nerve* comes ultimately from Greek *neuron = bowstring,* and it is certain that the Greeks strung their bows with tendons, not nerves.) The English *womb,* now applied only to the uterus, in the sixteenth century could also mean *abdomen, stomach* or *intestine.* Its more specific meaning may have arisen from its use as a euphemism for the female reproductive apparatus, just as *loins, reins* and *thigh* are Biblical euphemisms for the male genitalia.

Much English anatomic terminology shows the same tendency to apply metaphorically the names of common things that we shall see in Latin and Greek in the next chapter. In fact, many anatomic terms like *canal, chamber, column, floor, vault, wall* are simply translations of the corresponding Latin ones. *Eardrum* is a literal rendering of Greek *tympanon.* The *calf* of the leg was so named because it resembles the belly of a calf. Though etymologists are divided as to the origin of *kidney,* some believe it means *belly-egg.* In the nomenclature of microscopic anatomy and pathology we find figurative expressions of more recent adoption, such as *goblet, sickle* and *target* cells.

Names of common symptoms, and of diseases that were recognized before the era of scientific medicine, are usually English words: *ache, measles, sore, wound.*

Cough, croup and *hiccup* are onomatopoetic or echoic words—that is, their sounds are meant to imitate the sounds of the things they represent. The *whoop* of *whooping cough* (originally *hooping cough*) is another example. *Cough* is from Anglo-Saxon *cohhian; croup* from Danish *hropja. Hiccup* was spelled *hicket* or *hickock* when it first appeared in the sixteenth century. *Hiccough* is a venerable but erroneous variant spelling, by analogy with *cough. Spit* is derived from Anglo-Saxon *spaetan,* and *sputum* from Latin *spuere,* but there can be little doubt that both verbs go back to a common echoic Aryan root. Strange to say, *gargle* is not an instance of onomatopoeia, but is derived from French *gargouille=throat,* as is *gargoyle.*

The list also includes many compound words: *chillblain, frostbite, harelip, headache, smallpox* (2), *wryneck.* As in anatomy, the physician may find it necessary to substitute terms coined from the classic languages for native names of symptoms or diseases whose range of meanings is too broad. For instance, a patient who says he is *dizzy* may be complaining of ataxia, disorientation, restlessness, somnolence or vertigo. *Numbness* can mean anesthesia, hypesthesia, paresthesia or muscular weakness.

Stye is a modern spelling of *styan,* from still older Anglo-Saxon *stighende=a rising.* Both this word and the term for a pigpen were formerly spelled with a terminal *e.* Once customarily dropped from both words, the *e* has lately been revived to distinguish the medical term from the agricultural one. *Hangnail* is not quite what it seems: Anglo-Saxon *angnaegl* is a compound of *ang=pain* and *naegl=nail.*

Jaundice is old French *jaunisse=yellowness.* The *d* was inserted by the same natural process that put the *d* in *thunder* (Anglo-Saxon *thunor*). Like the *p* that often creeps into the pronunciation of *something,* this *d* sound seems to be called for by the phonetic pattern of English speech, and in *jaundice* and *thunder* it has become so universal that it is reflected in the spelling of the words.

Colic is a syncopated version of *colonic,* which entered the language directly from medical Latin around the thirteenth century in the sense of *a pain in the colon. Corn* comes from Latin *cornu=horn* by way of French, and is thus related to *cornea, corneum, cornification.*

A great many common English words for diseases and symptoms

---

2. So named to distinguish it from the *great pox* (syphilis). *Pox* is a phonetic spelling of *pocks,* from Anglo-Saxon *poc=pustule, ulcer.* Like *measles, pox* is singular when used as the name of a disease, plural when it refers to lesions, but for the latter application the spelling *pocks* is preferred. Though *cowpox* is a disease of cattle as well as man, *chickenpox* has nothing to do with chickens; the term is probably derived, a little irregularly, from Middle English *chiche=chick-pea,* from Latin *cicer.*

have died out of the vernacular, not because the diseases have been eradicated but because the layman's sophistication in language has kept pace with advances in medical science. *Ague* is an old-fashioned word borrowed from French *aigu,* which is cognate with our word *acute.* Though this term was once applied indiscriminately to any acute febrile illness, even the layman now recognizes that there is a difference between the common cold and an attack of malaria.

Squint, a borrowing from medieval Dutch *(schuinte = slope),* first appeared in English as *asquint* in about the fourteenth century. Originally *squint* meant *strabismus,* and it still has this significance in England. But as the word has acquired many figurative applications, and now means in American English *to look through narrowed eyelids,* the ophthalmologic connotation of the original word is quite lost to us.

Medical English preserves a few usages now considered archaic in the lay language: *great* toe, *gall*stone, *still*birth. Many other expressions have been borrowed by the physician from the common speech and given restricted, technical meanings. *Plague* is a French form of Latin *plaga = stroke, wound.* At first *plague* referred to a purely personal affliction, and only later was it applied to epidemics, perhaps because of its use to denominate the ten scourges called down by Moses on Egypt, as narrated in the Book of Exodus. *Plague* has disappeared from modern French, which preserves another derivative of the Latin word in its original strict sense: *plaie = wound.* In English, however, the word survives, and, through being applied to the various visitations of the Black Death to England and continental Europe in the sixteenth and seventeenth centuries, it has come to mean specifically the disease caused by *Pasteurella pestis.*

Migraine, too, is now the name of a specific disease, though when it came into English from French in the fifteenth century it meant merely a unilateral headache. It is a corruption (3) of Greek *hemicrania,* which is still used generically for any unilateral headache.

Orf is a shortened form of Anglo-Saxon *orfcwealm,* and like many abbreviations it retains the least important part of the original *(orf = cattle; cwealm = death, destruction,* related to modern *qualm).* Moreover, the current significance does not accord even with the part of the full expression that has been retained, for orf is a disease of sheep, which, though occasionally transmitted to humans, never afflicts cattle.

---

3. As we shall have occasion to use this word often, let us make it clear at the outset that a *corruption* is a variant, generally phonetic, whose derivation did not follow any established pattern of word formation. There is no derogation implied in the term, and no reproach attached to the use of "corrupt" forms.

Sick (from Anglo-Saxon *seoc*) was long the standard English adjective for *diseased* or *unwell*, but around the beginning of this century it began to give way to *ill*, a Scandinavian import that seems to have come in at the time of the Danish invasion. This change took place first in England, where *sick* had acquired the specific meaning of *vomiting or about to vomit*, a significance that it still preserves there. In recent years, *ill* has pretty much replaced *sick* in this country, too, and though we do not restrict the meaning of the latter word to persons suffering from nausea, we seem to regard it as a low or vulgar expression for which *ill* is a more refined substitute.

A number of English expressions have special denotations in medicine that are not generally appreciated or understood outside the profession: *shock, heart failure, soft tissues.* In professional use *strain* and *sprain* have specific and distinct meanings, as have *stammer* and *stutter.* Many words have been assigned special significations in the terminology of psychoanalysis: *conversion, insight, projection, sublimation.*

Most technical words referring to modern diagnosis and therapy had to be coined at the time when the diagnostic procedure or therapeutic technique was developed. The more recently this has occurred, the more likely is the term to have been made up of classic Latin or Greek stock instead of from English. *Salve* (from Anglo-Saxon *sealf* = *clarified butter*) has given way to the more genteel-sounding *ointment* (from Latin *unguentum*). *Draft* and *powder* have faded out because drugs are now seldom administered in these forms. Once very much in vogue, these terms were often qualified with not-very-illuminating adjectives *(black draft)* or named after the originator of the drug *(Dover's powder)* or its place of origin *(Seidlitz powder).*

Lozenge, which rhymes with *orange* though often mispronounced *lozenger,* comes from Provençal *losange.* Derived ultimately from Latin *laudare* = *to praise,* this word was first applied to tombstones bearing words of eulogy, then to roofing slates cut in the same general shape, and finally to anything else so formed. *Laudanum,* the old word for tincture of opium, is not from *laudare* but is a corruption of Greek *ladanon* = *gum, resin.*

Few surgical procedures in use today have common English names. An exception is *grafting.* Old French *greffe* (from Greek *graphein* = *to write*) meant *a stylus or pen,* and was applied figuratively to the scion or shoot of a tree inserted in another stock. In English this horticultural technique was therefore called *graffing* or *grafting,* and by a further extension of the metaphor this term has been applied in the modern era to surgical procedures in which living tissue is moved from one site to another. The name of the surgical *sound* is a figurative allusion to the depth-gauge used in navigation, which gets its name from Danish *sund* =*straits or shoals;* compare *Long Island Sound.*

Splint is a Dutch word, cognate with *spline* and *splinter,* and *stent* (a corruption of *extend*) in Middle English meant a stick used by a butcher to hold open a carcase. *Stupe* goes back at least as far as the fourteenth century and is derived from Latin *stupa*=*flannel.*

Even though the medical profession seems generally compelled to name every new thing with a fresh coinage from Latin or Greek, several modern concepts are expressed technically by good old Anglo-Saxon words: friction *rub, frozen* section, serum *sickness, heart block, slit* lamp.

No possible subject of discussion can be considered altogether taboo in the physician's consulting room, but certain words are so considered. Patterns of polite or proper usage among both laymen and physicians are often erratic. In neither group is *snot* or *puke* regarded as polite speech, yet *spit, belch* and *belly* are used by both without hesitation. Physicians may say *crotch, armpit* or *scab* in speaking to patients, but never among themselves, though there is no technical term whatever that is exactly equivalent to *scab.*

Whereas the fastidious nonprofessional is also careful to avoid both *gut* and *guts* except in figurative expressions ("A gut issue"; "The kid's got guts"), the physician freely uses the singular form as a generic term for the intestine (Anglo-Saxon *gutta*=*channel,* from *geotan*=*to pour*).

Which words are considered crude or vulgar or impolite is of course entirely a matter of custom and convention. It is doubtful that many of Chaucer's contemporaries were offended by his mentioning in the Prologue to *The Wife of Bath's Tale* that "Xantippa caste pisse upon his [Socrates'] heed," or by this line in *The Reeve's Tale:* "This Nicholas anon let fle a fart." Yet in America in the nineteenth century, *leg, breast* and even *woman* were considered obscenities, not to be pronounced before female company in any context whatever.

Stool has a long history of use in English as a euphemism for *feces.* A *close stool* was a sort of toilet chair equipped with an earthenware vessel under the seat, and in time *stool* came to be applied metaphorically to the act of defecation, a significance preserved in our expression *straining at stool.* Eventually the word was extended to the feces themselves.

Gas is neither Romance nor Anglo-Saxon nor Greek. In fact, the word did not exist until the seventeenth century, when it was coined by the Belgian monk and physician Jan van Helmont. Because it supplied a need in the language of chemistry and physics, it spread immediately to every civilized country and was assumed into all languages, soon appearing in derivative forms like *gaseous* and *gasoline.* It is used by physician and layman alike in this country for intestinal flatus, though the British prefer *wind.*

Space will not permit a thorough comparison of British and American medical usage, but a few differences may be mentioned in passing. What an American calls his *crazy bone* is an Englishman's *funny bone.* In England a lunatic is not *crazy* but *mad,* and an irate person is not *mad* but *angry.* The well-bred Englishman has a deeply rooted aversion to the word *bloody;* instead of a *bloody nose* he gets a *nosebleed.* An English woman in labor most assuredly does not experience a *bloody show,* and an English physician with any sense of propriety does not ask a nurse to change a *bloody dressing. Stomach,* in its broad, lay significance of *the abdomen,* is likewise taboo in polite speech in Britain, where a staid and sober middle-aged patient with abdominal pain solemnly informs the doctor that his *tummy* hurts.

An Englishman goes not to the *toilet* but to the *W. C.* or the *loo.* In England and Canada a *napkin* is either a baby's diaper or what we call a *sanitary napkin;* the Englishman dines with a *serviette* in his lap. What we know as *adhesive tape* is in England *sticking-plaster.* Not so many years ago the usual term there was *court plaster,* an allusion to the seventeenth-century custom according to which ladies of fashion appeared at court with patches of black sticking-plaster on their faces. Supposedly these patches were an enhancement of beauty, but it seems more likely that they served mainly to distract the eye of the beholder from plain features, and no doubt in many instances also to conceal pimples.

In England a physician graduates with the degree of Bachelor of Medicine (M.B.), though he may pursue further study and eventually earn an M.D. In either case he is addressed as "doctor," and *Dr.* is placed before his name unless he happens to be a surgeon. Whether a surgeon has a doctoral degree or not, custom demands that he be called *Mr.* This curious practice, still very strictly observed, dates back to the days when bloodletting, incision of abscesses, and other cutting procedures were performed by barbers rather than by members of the medical profession.

It would be remarkable if a language as colorful and flexible as English had not given birth to some highly picturesque expressions even in the technical terminology of a scientific discipline. Most medical terms of this sort, like the anatomic metaphors *calf* and *eardrum* already mentioned, are figurative in origin.

The history of the passage of a word or root through time is often not so much a record of its movement from one language to another as a tracing of its metaphoric extensions. For example, Aryan *bhogo* and its Greek descendant *phogo* had a very definite and concrete meaning: *to cook.* (Our *bake* is a modern derivative in the Germanic branch of the family.) But the related Latin noun *focus* was applied to both the kitchen hearth and the *fire,* whence the modern Spanish and Italian words for fire, *fuego* and *fuoco.*

The next step in the metaphoric evolution of *focus* was its use to denominate *a device used to start a fire,* a burning-glass. In 1604, when the astronomer Kepler needed a word for *the point at which light rays converge after passing through a lens,* he chose this figurative expression. Subsequently it was extended to a broad range of other applications in geometry, astronomy and optics, and the verb *to focus* was born.

By still further extension of meaning, this verb began to be used with instruments in which there was no convergence of rays (as in a slide projector) or even no lens (as in a television receiver). Nowadays it is used in a purely abstract way, as when we say we are *focussing our attention* on the liver, or *focussing our efforts* on prevention. Meanwhile, the sense of the original noun has evolved, along another track, to *center or source,* as in *focus of infection* and *unifocal emboli.*

Focus is an example of what philologists call a dead metaphor—one whose figurative meaning has replaced its literal one. Dead metaphors need not originate as foreign words. The literal meaning of *brand* is *something burnt.* Though this sense is still familiar to cattle ranchers and devotees of the western, most people nowadays think of a brand as a *trade name,* and in many instances the meaning has been carried further. On the one hand, it is often concretized, as when we speak of a brand as *the product of a particular manufacturer,* and on the other hand it may be further abstracted, as when we say we don't like somebody's *brand of humor.*

In his efforts to apply accurate and intelligible designations to abnormal appearances, sounds, odors and sensible phenomena generally, the physician has often had recourse to metaphor and simile. It takes no very creative intellect to fabricate an expression like *air hunger, rusty sputum,* or *napkin-ring obstruction.* Moreover, as these are vivid, explicit and readily understandable, they require no laborious memorization.

Abnormal configurations and movements are accurately depicted by terms like *bamboo spine, clubfoot, cogwheel rigidity, collar-button abscess, cotton-wool exudate, flame hemorrhage, green-stick fracture, hammer toe, hare-lip, hilar dance, mallet finger, moth-eaten lung, pill-rolling tremor, saddle nose, silver fork deformity, spider angioma* and *staghorn calculus.*

Sounds, too, are often called by picturesque names such as *cracked-*

pot resonance, gallop rhythm, machinery and *seagull murmurs, musical rales* and *pistol-shot pulse.* A somewhat farfetched metaphor is *diamond-shaped murmur,* referring to the visual representation of the crescendo and decrescendo of this murmur on the phonocardiogram. Even smells may acquire figurative names like the *fruity* breath of diabetic ketosis and the *mousy* odor of pharyngeal diphtheria.

A remarkable number of descriptive figures refer to food and drink. Consider, as a representative and most unappetizing sample, *oat-cell* carcinoma, the *branny desquamation* of scarlatina and the *rice-water stools* of cholera; the *mulberry molars* of congenital syphilis, the *currant-jelly stools* of intussusception, the *strawberry hemangioma,* the *strawberry tongue* of scarlatina and the *strawberry gallbladder* of choles-terolosis; the *potato nodes* of sarcoidosis and the *bread-and-butter heart* of fibrinous pericarditis; the *apple-jelly lesion* of lupus vulgaris; the *maple-syrup urine* of cystinosis and the *Coca-Cola urine* of acute glomerulone-phritis; *chocolate cysts, coffee-grounds emesis, chicken-fat clots, port-wine stain, caseous necrosis* and *milk-leg.*

Though dead metaphors are uncommon in medical speech, some current expressions are based on comparisons that mean little to the modern physician. The *water-hammer pulse* of aortic insufficiency is named not after a piece of machinery, as many think, but after a child's toy. A water hammer is a large glass cylinder, closed at both ends and partly filled with water. The air is exhausted before the cylinder is sealed, and when the toy is repeatedly inverted end over end, the water slams back and forth all in a mass because it need not displace any air to do so. One wonders how many pathologists who speak glibly of *nutmeg* and *hobnail* livers have ever seen the cut surface of a whole nutmeg, or a leather boot-sole studded over with round-headed nails.

A few English descriptive terms are so fanciful as to verge upon the poetic. Such, for example, are *joint mice, kissing ulcers, proudflesh* (which goes back to the fourteenth century), the *ripe cataract* (or *cervix*), the *sentinel pile* and *silent gallstones.* The vernacular has provided a few vivid and colorful expressions like *knock knee* and *wisdom tooth,* which are used even by physicians, and *trick knee, goose pimples,* and *a frog in the throat,* which are not.

In turn, a few medical expressions have become figures of speech in the lay language: *blind spot, jaundiced eye,* an *atrophied* conscience, a *rash* of bad checks.

𝔄𝔡𝔧𝔢𝔠𝔱𝔦𝔳𝔢𝔰

Some languages have adjectived more.

John Horne Tooke
Epea Pteroenta, or The Diversions of Purley

As we have already seen, modern English has discarded most of the inflectional system of Anglo-Saxon. It has also largely dispensed with certain patterns of affixation that were common even as recently as the eighteenth century. We do not, for instance, insist any longer upon the ending *–en (–n)* to indicate that a noun like *wood* or *leather* has been turned into an adjective: *wooden, leathern.* Indeed, one of the features that makes English such a succinct and economical language is its freedom in using nouns as adjectives without any change in form, as in *bone* metastasis, *nerve* deafness, *sickle cell* anemia, and *blood vessel disease patient care data selection* process.

Some have endeavored to explain this usage by pointing to the fact that many English words do not form adjectives. According to this view, we say *heart disease* because the nearest adjective to *heart* is the Greek-derived *cardiac,* and *wound dehiscence* because there is no adjective in the language that means *pertaining to a wound* except *vulnery* and *woundy,* both obsolete and the latter profane as well.

But the unavailability of adjectives formed from native English material is just as likely to be the result as the cause of the practice of using nouns as adjectives. Even when an adjective is readily available, we often use a noun form instead: *bile* pigment, *sex* differentiation, *virus* infection (4). Only occasionally is there any cogent reason for doing so, as when we say *rectus spasm* to avoid the confusion that might be engendered by *rectal spasm.*

The headline or telegram style of forming compound expressions is a characteristic of all Germanic languages, in contrast to the Romance and the Slavic, which do not use it at all. German freely runs together three or four nouns to form a single word of twenty-five or more letters. Though in English compounds of ancient vintage we may find the component words joined together in this fashion *(gallbladder, headache, pinworm),* more often they stand apart *(lung abscess, skin graft, sedimentation rate).* A hyphen is rare except to denote different degrees or planes

---

4. It will be noted that many of the words and expressions cited throughout the rest of the chapter are not native English in any sense. We are now concerned not so much with words that are structurally or historically English as with the dynamics of the language as a medium of technical communication.

of modification: we write *liver cell* but *liver-cell injury; rat bite* but *rat-bite fever.*

Neither French nor Russian can translate any of these phrases without either inserting a preposition between the nouns *(ache of the head)* or turning one of them into a formal adjective *(pulmonary abscess).* Though this may seem a deficiency in these languages, it has its practical advantages; the English custom of using a noun as an adjective without somehow signalling the hearer or reader that there has been a change in the role of the word gives rise to an incalculable amount of confusion.

To appreciate this fully we must examine a second peculiarity of modern English, especially technical English, with respect to the adjective. We all learned in school that "an adjective is a word that describes or limits a noun or pronoun," but this definition is defective as applied to the *English* adjective, because it does not take into account two variant constructions almost unique in our language.

In one of these, an adjective complements the noun by indicating the object of an action expressed by the noun. Thus, *ligation of the tubes* becomes *tubal ligation,* and *resection of a segment* becomes *segmental resection.* It is ironic that a language which readily presses nouns into service as adjectives *(spine films)* should so often insist upon making a formal adjective out of a noun that is actually functioning as a noun, that is, as the object of an action *(spinal fusion).*

But the English adjective is often forced into a role that is still more enigmatic. Speakers of most modern languages would never think of saying, "He is under observation for suspected leukemia"; they would refer to "suspicion of leukemia." They would regard as a semantic absurdity the statement that "The patient died of a probable myocardial infarction." Here, as in the preceding example, the adjective modifies the meaning of the whole sentence instead of just the noun to which it is formally appended. The adverbial nature of its function can be more clearly seen when the sentence is recast in a more logical form: "He died, probably of a myocardial infarction."

Medical English is full of statements like this one: "In protracted cases of asthma, the physician must be prepared to treat possible acute congestive failure." A Spaniard or a Pole trying to decipher this sentence might well wonder what *possible acute congestive failure* is, how it differs from the ordinary kind, how it is treated, and whether there is an *impossible acute congestive failure* as well.

When more than one of these peculiarly English uses of the adjective are operative in the formation of a sentence, the resulting construction is often ambiguous or obscure. *Hypokalemic conduction defect* and *interventricular conduction defect* look like parallel constructions at first glance, but upon analysis they prove to have entirely different internal relations. The first means *a defect, caused by hypokalemia, of conduction;* the second, *a defect of interventricular conduction.* That is, in the first example the first adjective modifies *conduction,* and in the second it modifies *defect.* The long-established *coronary artery disease* and the brash new-comer *coronary heart disease* compose another such pair. When a patient is advised to avoid *oily hair preparations,* does that mean he should avoid hair preparations that are oily, or preparations that are for oily hair? If *iron* and *tendon* are adjectives in *iron nails* and *tendon reflexes,* what are they in *iron deficiency* and *tendon transplant?* Grammarians might debate this question until the end of time and not reach unanimity.

The liberal and sometimes illogical extension of function of the English adjective is perhaps less often productive of genuinely ambiguous than of awkward and tedious prose. The reader of a piece of writing that is heavily encumbered with such constructions is like a traveller in a strange city, who must stop at every corner and scan the street signs before proceeding. His progress is slow, he makes false starts along wrong streets, and he may end up completely lost. Sometimes the uniquely English conventions governing the use of the adjective result in syntactic irregularities that are altogether indefensible because they do not mean what they say. For instance, in "Staphylococci are among the most common bacteria that cause septic arthritis" there can be little doubt that what the writer really means is "Staphylococci are among *the bacteria that most commonly cause* septic arthritis."

Much less likely to generate confusion is the practice of converting formal adjectives into nouns. Most languages can make absolutes out of adjectives; Plato discoursed in Greek of *the true, the good,* and *the beautiful,* and Napoleon went in French from *the sublime* to *the ridiculous.* But English is especially apt to employ adjectives substantively, as in *a pelvic* [*examination*], the [*membrana*] *mucosa, the lymphatic* [*channel*]s, *a coronary* [*occlusion*], *an antibiotic* [*drug*], the [*nervus*] *vagus.*

In *adrenal suppression, antibiotic therapy, protozoan disease* and *rectal glove,* words that were originally adjectives and have evolved into nouns while preserving their adjectival endings *(–al, –an, –ic)* now operate once again as adjectives, but with significant difference in meaning. Consider, for example, the distinction between *rectal* when applied to *polyp* (primary adjectival sense) and when applied to *glove* (secondary sense, derived from use of the word as a noun; *i.e., rectal examination*).

The persistence of adjectival endings in words that have become nouns occasionally has peculiar results. In *subarachnoid hemorrhage* the ending *–oid* is made to do double duty, and no additional adjectival ending is applied to the noun *arachnoid*. In analogous expressions involving nouns that do not have adjectival endings, the endings are always supplied: *subdural, subperiosteal hemorrhage.*

Verbs

The verb is the most highly condensed and the most highly abstract element of discourse.

Frederick Bodmer
The Loom of Language (5)

Verbs represent almost the last degree of refinement in the development of language. We do very well without them in such expressions as "No kidding?" "Me neither," "Merry Christmas," "Never a dull moment," "Why the long face?" and "Strike three like hell!" Though a traveler in a foreign country must know many nouns, perhaps two or three hundred, to communicate with people who do not speak English, he needs only three verbs: *to be, to go* and *to want.* But there have been verbs in all the Aryan languages as far back as scholars can trace them, and though it is likely that most words that now function as verbs were originally nouns, the only support we have for that thesis is the fact that the process of forming verbs from nouns (6) has been going on since the beginning of written language and continues to this day.

A noun may be used as a verb in English without any change in form *(to curette, to biopsy, to gastroscope)* or a verb may be fashioned from a noun by addition of a suffix *(digitalize, cannulate, cornify).* A large class of verbs has been manufactured by the process known as back-formation, in which a suffix is *removed* from a noun to yield what looks as though it ought to be the verb from which the noun was formed.

Physicians are especially prone to fabricate verbs in this fashion from Greek nouns ending in *–osis: anastomose, ankylose, cyanose, ecchymose, fibrose, metamorphose, necrose, osmose, sclerose, stenose, thrombose.* Though some of the verbs in this list are considered a little more acceptable than others, they are all in common use in the spoken language of medicine. Other nouns that are especially fruitful sources of back-formations are

5. Bodmer F: THE LOOM OF LANGUAGE. New York, W W Norton, 1944
6. And *vice versa.* Nearly every English noun ending in *–ment (government, establishment),* *–ion (revision, seduction)* or *–sis (analysis, emphasis)* has been formed from a verb in one language or another.

those ending in *–esis (diapedese, diaphorese, diurese, electrophorese)* and *–ion (counteragress, infarct, percuss).*

All verbs created by back-formation are considered illegitimate, because the process implies an erroneous belief that the resulting verb actually existed before the noun on which the operation is performed. But there is certainly nothing illogical about looking for a verb in such a word as *measurement* or *lysis.* As we have noted, nearly all such nouns are derived from verbs. But whereas *measurement* was probably formed in English from *measure,* no English verb corresponds to the noun *lysis.* We are therefore faced with the alternatives of using the original Greek verb with all its two-hundred-odd inflexional forms *(luo, luso, elusa, leluka, lelumai, elelumen, eluthen,* etc., etc., etc.) or of fashioning an English verb: *lyse, lysed, lysing.*

Some have objected to the expression *to debride* on the grounds that it is derived by back-formation from the French noun *débridement.* But though English can and readily does borrow French nouns bodily, since they are uninflected except for plural endings, French verbs cannot be handled correctly without a knowledge of the language. The use of *debride, debrided, debriding* is thus justified by practical considerations if not by formal linguistic principles.

The case of *to curette* is somewhat different. The noun was coined in French around the fifteenth century from the verb *curer=to cleanse* (compare modern French *cure-dents=toothpick*), but it was only at the end of the nineteenth century that the noun *curetage* (note the spelling) appeared in French medical literature and was taken into English. Whether we look upon our verb *to curette* as a back-formation from *curettage* (American spelling) or as a noun employed without change of form as a verb, it is obviously a better choice than *cure.*

Whatever opinion philologists may entertain of them, some back-formations *(diagnose, donate, edit, legislate)* have lived down the irregularity of their birth to become perfectly respectable. The rest run the gamut from the acceptable *(percuss, anastomose)* to the vulgar *(replete, diaphorese).* What makes an acceptable form acceptable is that it expresses a certain idea more clearly than any other single word with a better title to existence. The vulgarisms either are superfluous variants of established words *(replete* for *replenish,* by false analogy with *deplete)* or express an idea for which a simpler word exists *(diaphorese* for *sweat* or, if you must have two syllables, *perspire).*

Verbs created by any of these processes may occasionally become a source of confusion if they happen to be identical with words already in the language. Many English verbs that began life as nouns are still a little awkward in their new occupation. When a surgeon *drains* an abscess he *establishes drainage* (primary meaning of the verb) but when he *drains* a cholecystectomy he *inserts a drain* (noun used as a verb). *To cycle* can mean *to ride a bicycle* or *to establish regular menses*. *To type* a specimen of blood is not the same thing as *to type* the laboratory report. *To dust* may mean either to remove dust or to apply it. In modern parlance, *to cast* an extremity means *to apply a cast*. Logically the past tense and past participle should be formed with *–ed*, but because the original verb *cast* (the parent of all other English *casts* literal and metaphorical) is irregular and does not change in the past tenses, we hear and read "The leg was cast." An analogous usage is seen in "He was cast as a villain."

Microorganisms treated with formalin are said to be *formalized;* there is, however, a considerably older word of the same form in the language of business, law and diplomacy with an altogether different meaning. A patient treated with anticoagulant is said to be *anticoagulated,* an expression whose formation includes more than one linguistic irregularity. But as the term is well established and is understood perfectly by those who hear or read it in the course of their professional activities, only a rigid formalist or a lunatic would opt for a theoretically more logical form such as *anticoagulatantized.*

Back-formations, too, sometimes come into conflict with established words. *Incinerate* means *to reduce to ashes,* and a trash burner is therefore called an *incinerator.* By back-formation a new verb has been manufactured from *incinerator* which happens to be identical in form with the original but very different in meaning. In the familiar warning, "Do not puncture or incinerate can," *incinerate* means not *to reduce to ashes* but *to put into an incinerator.*

Yet it is sometimes just because it does introduce a new shade of meaning that a back-formation may gain a foothold and become acceptable. *Obligate,* once a vulgar and superfluous variant of *oblige,* now has an application that distinguishes it from the latter word and so seems to entitle it to a separate existence. In "The General Assembly declined to obligate funds for new hospital construction," *oblige* could not possibly be substituted for its upstart cousin.

At first glance we are likely to characterize such verbs as *go, walk,* and *run* as irrevocably intransitive, since the actions they denote cannot logically have an object. Yet in the expressions *go your way, walk the dog,* and *run an errand,* these verbs take on a transitive character. A similar process can affect technical terms. The primitive meaning of *abort* is *to miscarry* or *to fail to develop,* a sense in which it is exclusively intransitive. Nowadays, though, we speak of "aborting a migraine headache" in a fashion that clearly shows that the verb is thought of as transitive.

Another example is *adhere,* formerly confined to intransitive applications like "Fragments of cerumen may adhere to the tympanic membrane." Yet now we often hear and read such statements as "The graft was adhered to the prepared site."

These changes follow well-established patterns of linguistic evolution, and no one could reasonably object to them on the grounds that such verbs are unintelligible in their new applications. In fact, this kind of functional evolution is yet another instance of the almost unique tendency of the English language to diversify the function of a word without changing its form.

3

our classical heritage

Latin

Latin is a dead language, as dead as it can be;
First it killed the Romans, and now it's killing me.

Schoolboy's jeremiad

According to tradition, the city of Rome was founded by the Latians or Latins in 753 B.C. Though they were the ancestors of the Italian race, the Latins were not the only inhabitants of Italy in those ancient days, nor even the most numerous. The founders of Rome shared a common ethnic origin with the far more widespread Umbrians, whose languages, Umbrian and Oscan, were closely related to Latin. By contrast, the Etruscans were originally immigrants from Asia Minor who colonized the district of Italy known as Etruria (modern Tuscany) around the tenth century before Christ, and grew wealthy through their skill in metalworking. The Etruscan language, of which written records date from as far back as 800 B.C., is still largely a riddle to scholars.

Neither the Umbrians nor the Latins had an alphabet of their own. The Umbrians eventually borrowed the alphabet of the Etruscans, but the Latins got theirs—essentially the one in which this book is printed (1)—from some Greek colonists at Cumae. (According to an alternate theory, the Greek alphabet passed through the hands of the Etruscans to the Latins.) Having acquired a system of writing, the Latins lost no time in putting it to use: the oldest surviving remnants of their language were chiseled in stone before 500 B.C.

By the middle of the second century B.C., Rome had conquered

---

1. It had no g, w or y, and made no distinction between i and j or between u and v. There were symbols for th, ph and ch, but as primitive Latin had no such sounds the symbols were dropped. They do survive in the "Roman" numerals for 50, 100 and 1000, which though now written L, C and M are not really derived from these letters but are corruptions of the discarded compound consonants.

Greece and Carthage and was well on her way to world dominion. She already had a rich literature, which would reach its full flower during the Augustan Age (31 B.C. to 14 A.D.) in the exquisite verses of Horace, Virgil and Ovid.

As we have already observed in Chapter 1, it is doubtful that the Latin language as preserved in the works of these classical authors was ever a medium of common speech. Classic Latin was the language of taste and refinement and culture, the language of epic poems and legal edicts and long orations composed at leisure. But it was the common speech, or Vulgar Latin, that broke up into what we call the Romance languages during the Dark Ages, losing its own identity in the process.

If Latin had survived only in the works of the classical Roman writers, it is unlikely that it would have survived at all, and fairly certain that it would not have become the universal medium of scholarship many centuries after the fall of the Roman Empire. But it must be remembered that in the first and second centuries A.D., Rome was the center not only of western civilization but also of Christianity, and Latin was adopted as the official language of the new faith. While the spoken language disintegrated and evolved, the written language remained nearly static, embalmed in the works of the early Fathers of the Church. Towards the end of the fourth century St. Jerome prepared a Latin translation of the Sacred Scriptures, the so-called Vulgate edition. Christian missionaries, starting with St. Augustine at Canterbury in 597, carried the Latin language into Britain and first taught the Anglo-Saxons to write. It was at this early period that a few Latin terms associated with religion entered the Anglo-Saxon tongue, *e.g. minster* (from *monasterium*) and *bishop* (from *episcopus*).

But it is not with ecclesiastical Latin, nor yet with the second and much greater accession of Romance words into English by way of Norman French, that we are here concerned. During the Dark Ages, Latin was the possession of the priests and monks, who together with a few secular scholars represented the literate minority. Though these men could read the works of the Augustan poets with ease, the Latin in which they daily wrote and taught, argued and joked, was a debased form of the classic language, which we know as "dog-Latin." More limited in vocabulary than the Latin of Virgil or Horace, dog-Latin was augmented with many vulgarisms and borrowings from other languages; the monks were not above taking a Gothic or Arabic word and Latinizing it by tacking on a Latin ending.

The Renaissance brought about a remarkable revival of the Latin language and its literature. All the classical writings that had survived the Dark Ages were republished, edited, analyzed and commented upon by a whole new race of classical scholars. A knowledge of Latin became not only a key to the door of learning but a means of communication among scholars across the length and breadth of the civilized world.

In medieval universities from Oxford to Buda, from Uppsala to Florence, Latin was the language of textbooks, lectures, recitations and examinations. Academic and medieval Latin has left its mark on all modern European languages, including English. *Gaudy,* originally applied to the nocturnal carousings of students, is derived from the medieval drinking song *Gaudeamus igitur.* We still call a patent medicine or quack remedy a *nostrum;* each band of traveling mountebanks (many of them medical school dropouts) referred to the panacea they hawked from town to town as "our own *(nostrum)* secret formula." The phrases for which our abbreviations *a.m., p.m., etc., i.e.* and *e.g.* stand are pure Latin, as are such words as *alibi, bonus, gratis, medium, posse, quorum, stet* and *via.*

Latin also became the language of jurisprudence, and a great many modern legal terms are Latin, some of them dating back even to Roman times and the legal system first codified under the emperor Justinian in the CORPUS JURIS CIVILIS (529–535 A.D.): *corpus delicti, habeas corpus, nolo contendere, prima facie, res ipsa loquitur.* One such phrase, *in re=* [*facts*] *in the case* [*of*], often appears at the head of a medical report, and *re* is sometimes loosely used as an abbreviation for the preposition *regarding.*

The development of printing from movable type led to a remarkable spread of literacy throughout the civilized world. Though only the sons of the wealthy received formal educations in the liberal arts or were prepared for careers in law or medicine, nearly all boys were instructed in the rudiments of reading and writing. English elementary education from the sixteenth to the nineteenth century was largely a matter of mastering Latin grammar and perusing the works of the great Latin authors.

Henry VIII and his daughter Elizabeth I were both fluent in Latin. The syntactic structure of English had scarcely been analyzed in their day; when a grammar was finally formulated for this extraordinary hybrid of Teutonic and French, this language that had virtually dispensed with inflections and relied upon word order to indicate functional relationships among the elements of a sentence, it was but the Latin grammar remodeled and recast.

An immense number of new English words were framed from Latin during the post-Renaissance period. Some of these fabrications no doubt satisfied definite needs, but a great many others were invented by writers who sought to produce erudite-sounding English prose and who knew that almost anyone who could read at all would be able to decipher coinages from Latin. Some few of these coinages took hold and became a permanent part of the language. No one is certain when and how such words as *position, gravity* and *solid* first entered English —whether from French during Norman times or directly from Latin after the revival of classical learning.

Many of the coinages affected by English scholars during the sixteenth and seventeenth centuries were not so straightforward as these. The works of Roger Ascham, Latin tutor to Queen Elizabeth I; Thomas Browne, physician and author of RELIGIO MEDICI; and Francis Bacon, statesman and essayist, are studded with impromptu coinages as well as "learned" words now long out of use, such as are absolutely unintelligible to anyone without a knowledge of Latin. Their contemporary, the rhetorician Sir Thomas Wilson, objected to words of this kind as "inkhorn terms," an epithet that has stuck.

In the eighteenth century Samuel Johnson, the compiler of the first comprehensive dictionary of English and the greatest philologist of his day, had a reputation for clouding an issue by substituting several sesquipedalian words coined wholesale from Latin or Greek when one plain English word of a syllable or two would do. In his DICTIONARY OF THE ENGLISH LANGUAGE ON HISTORICAL PRINCIPLES (1755), he defined *network* as "anything reticulated or decussated, at equal distances, with interstices between the intersections." It is hard to imagine that anyone capable of deriving information from this definition would be ignorant of the meaning of the word defined!

Like native English words, coinages from Latin often change in meaning with the passage of time. When Desdemona remarks that Othello will "return incontinent," she is not predicting that her husband will develop bladder trouble; *incontinent* meant *immediately* in Shakespeare's day.

Latin did not die out suddenly as a medium of scholarship in the English-speaking world, but some idea of when it began to wane in importance may be gathered from these historical facts: 1) When Sir Thomas More wrote UTOPIA in 1516, he composed the work in Latin and left it that way. English translations were made by others; none was printed until 1551, sixteen years after More's death. 2) In 1597 Sir Francis Bacon issued the first set of his ESSAYS. Though he wrote and published them in English, he took care to prepare a Latin translation, now lost, in order that they might be preserved for posterity in a language of more permanence than English. 3) Robert Burton wanted to publish his ANATOMY OF MELANCHOLY in Latin, but no publisher would take the chance that enough readers of Latin would buy it, and he was obliged to bring it out, in 1621, in English.

As the physical sciences gradually separated themselves from the welter of superstition that had surrounded the phenomena of nature during the Dark Ages, they began to develop and differentiate into mathematics, physics, chemistry and biology. The universal language of science, as of letters, was Latin. Scientists and scholars even Latinized their names. Thus the Italian Gabriello Fallopio and the Frenchman François de la Boe became Fallopius and Sylvius. A few invented Latin names for themselves out of thin air, like the brilliant and enigmatic Swiss physician Paracelsus, whose real name was Theophrastus Bombastus von Hohenheim.

It was during the sixteenth century that the great bulk of Latin anatomic nomenclature was codified. Some terms dated back many centuries to Roman times, others were coined to denominate structures newly discovered. Though some of it has been supplanted in recent years by a more systematic nomenclature, much of this medieval Latin terminology lives on in daily use. Its characteristic feature is the metaphorical application of names of familiar objects to bodily structures of similar form.

Topographic and architectural features are recalled by such terms as *fornix = arch, fossa = ditch, pons = bridge* and *cloaca = sewer*. There are at least four *aqueducts* in the human body. Every part of the house is represented, from the *roof (tectum)* to the *cellars (antrum)*, from the *gate (porta* [2]*)* and *entry-hall (vestibulum)* to the *inner court (atrium)* and *living room (thalamus)*. The dining room supplies a *dish (patella)* and a *bowl (acetabulum)*, a *bottle (ampulla)* and a *cup (calyx)*. *Infundibulum* means *funnel;* indeed, the English word is a corruption of the Latin one.

The human body was a veritable zoo to the early anatomists, who found therein a *worm (vermis)* and a *snail (cochlea)*, a *cock's comb (crista galli)*, a *bird's claw (calcar avis)* and a *goose's foot (pes anserinus)*, and a host of *little mice (musculi)*. Not only is the *horse's tail (cauda equina)* present, but *bridle (frenum)*, *stirrup (stapes)* and *saddle (sella)* as well, and even the blacksmith's *hammer (malleus)* and *anvil (incus)*. [Other implements include a *plowshare (vomer)*, a *scythe (falx)* and an *olive-press (torcular)*.]

The vegetable kingdom is represented in *uvula = little grape, glans*

2. The term *porta hepatis = gate of the liver* has fallen into disuse, and so the original sense of *portal vein* is not so obvious as formerly. Still, one cannot help wondering at the extraordinary etymology according to which *portal* is sometimes derived from *portare = to carry*.

=nut, ramus=branch, cortex=bark, lens=seed, piriform=pear-shaped and *pisiform=pea-shaped.*

In their fondness for metaphor and simile anatomists have even gone so far as to name one part of the body after another. *Os cervicis* means literally *mouth of the neck. Capitellum, pedicle, ventricle, auricle,* and *lingula* are diminutives of words meaning respectively *head, foot, belly, ear* and *tongue.* Not all of these diminutives are strictly reasonable: the lingula of the left lung is considerably larger than the tongue.

Some comparisons have been a little overworked. The *coronal suture* of the skull lies, appropriately enough, across the *crown* of the head, and has given its name to the *coronal section* of descriptive anatomy. To the early anatomists the vasculature of that noble organ the heart looked like a crown, and they accordingly dubbed these vessels the *coronary arteries* and *veins.* The *coronary ligament* of the knee joint rests atop the tibia and around the semilunar cartilages, and with a little imagination can be said to crown them, just as the *coronary ligament* of the liver crowns that organ. The *corona* of the glans penis and the *crown* of a tooth nearly exhaust the list. *(Coronoid* is from Greek *korone=crow.)*

Many Latin anatomic terms are purely descriptive: *quadratus* and *rotundum* mean respectively *square* and *round* and are incidentally the originals of the English terms. *Rectus* and *rectum* mean *straight; vagus, wandering. Duodenum* refers to the length of the organ, which is *twelve* inches. *Innominate,* a rather whimsical designation, actually means *unnamed.*

Before the invention of the clock, the normal heartbeat was one of the most reliable measures of short intervals of time. Since in early days the pulse was taken at the side of the head, this area was called *tempus=time,* and our *temple* is a corruption of Latin *tempus* or *temporalis.* A great many other anatomic terms go all the way back to Roman times. *Abdomen* was in use in the second century B.C., and has been variously derived from *abdere=to hide away* and *adeps=fat. Testis* means *witness;* its use for the male gonad, which goes back at least to Horace's time, is probably derived from the primitive custom of taking an oath with a hand on the testicles. (Compare the ancient Hebrew practice noted in Genesis 24:3 and again in Genesis 47:29.) *Cadaver,* literally *one who has fallen,* is classic Latin for a *corpse* or *carcase.* The *os sacrum=holy bone* is so called, according to Monro (3), "from being offered as a dainty Bit in Sacrifice."

3. Monro, Alexander: THE ANATOMY OF THE HUMAN BONES, 3rd ed., 1741, as quoted in THE OXFORD ENGLISH DICTIONARY.

Mamma=breast is another very old word, which occurs in classic Greek as well as in Latin. Besides *mamma,* Latin and Greek used *papa* for *breast;* compare *papilla, papule,* and *pap.* These are examples of "baby words" taken into the formal language. Infants of all races begin speaking with the syllables *ma, pa, ta (da),* often repeated several times. In most Aryan languages the word for *mother* begins with *m* and the word for *father* with *p* (*f* or *v* in the Teutonic branch). In the first century B.C., by which time *mamma* already meant *breast* in literary Latin, the grammarian Varro recorded the fact that Roman children called their mothers *mamma* and their fathers *tata* (compare *dada, daddy*). In modern Rumanian the formal words for *mother* and *father* are *mama* and *tata.* French and German *tante=aunt* is a variant of *tata. Pupil* in both of its current English senses, the zoological term *pupa,* and French *poupée=doll* (whence *puppy*) are all variants of *papa.*

The Romans were not particularly exact in their use of everyday words to designate parts of the body. The science of medicine was practically unknown in Rome until the second century B.C., and even then almost the only physicians in Rome were Greeks or Egyptians. Accordingly, Latin anatomic terms did not acquire practical importance until comparatively late. *Brachium* could mean either *the whole arm* or just *the forearm. Uterus,* like English *womb,* had both a special significance, equivalent to that which it has in modern anatomy, and a more general one of *belly.* In the AENEID Virgil speaks of the *uterus* of the wooden horse of Troy, meaning its hollow interior.

Some words borrowed from classic Latin by the anatomist underwent shifts in significance during the Late Latin period, and appear in the Romance languages with other meanings. *Bucca,* which to the Romans of the pre-Christian era meant *cheek,* replaced *os* in Vulgar Latin as the usual word for *mouth,* so that *os* died childless, and the Romance languages use derivatives of *bucca* to mean *mouth:* Spanish and Italian *boca,* French *bouche.* But before it lost its strict anatomic meaning of *cheek, bucca* gave rise to two derivatives in classic Latin. One was the adjective *buccalis,* which survives in English in the homophones *buccal* and *buckle.* (The latter word was first applied to the fastening of the chin-strap of a helmet, which lay *along the cheek.*) *Buccina* was the name of a military trumpet whose sounding required vigorous use of the cheek muscles; from this word we have the anatomic term *buccinator.*

The classic Latin *crus=shin, leg* died out and was replaced by two other words in Vulgar Latin, both of them from Greek. *Perna,* originally signifying a *leg of pork,* a *ham,* appears unchanged in modern Portuguese, and as *pierna* in Spanish. Italian *gamba* and French *jambe* (whence our *ham*) came from Vulgar Latin *gamba,* a corruption of Greek *kampe = bend, joint.* In modern technical usage *crural* does not refer to the lower leg but rather to the thigh or the groin.

Some anatomic terms have been given more specific meanings in modern times than they had in the works of the medieval anatomists, though examples of the earlier usages may persist. Thus *ligamentum = something that binds* has nowadays a strict application to connective tissue bands that support and stabilize a joint, but instances of an older and more general significance survive in the *hepatic* and *uterine ligaments.*

From the early Middle Ages the developing science of medicine, like its ancillary disciplines of anatomy, chemistry and pharmacy, used Latin as the medium of communication. Hence it naturally came about that drug names were Latinized, and when the first British Pharmacopoeia was issued during Shakespeare's lifetime it was entirely in Latin. The physician's prescriptions, once extremely elaborate, were of course also written in Latin. Since in the sixteenth and seventeenth centuries any educated patient could have understood such prescriptions, and moreover since many men of leisure cultivated a knowledge of chemistry and botany, there is no reason to believe that physicians wrote in Latin, in those days at least, to keep their patients from knowing what medicine they were taking. Though it was just as true then as now that "a little learning is a dangerous thing," the useful "learning" of the physician was often just as "little" as that of his patient.

By the eighteenth century, prescription-writing had become a very complex and exacting art; a particularly accomplished practitioner might fill several pages in formulating a single concoction. Instructions to the patient were scarcely less elaborate than those to the pharmacist. As was inevitable, many of the elements of the prescription, having degenerated into ritual, came to be represented by abbreviations and symbols, many of which survive to this day.

Placebo is a Latin word meaning *I shall be pleasing,* which has come into medical parlance by a devious route. The last sentence (verse 9) of Psalm CXIV as given in the Vulgate is *"Placebo Domino in regione vivorum"*— "I shall be pleasing unto the Lord in the land of the living." This sentence was adopted as the opening of the Office for the Dead in the Latin Rite, and *placebo* later came to be a catchword for obsequiousness or servility. By the early nineteenth century it had acquired its modern meaning, "a medicine adapted more to please than benefit the patient (4)."

4. Hooper, Robert: MEDICAL DICTIONARY, 1811, as quoted in THE OXFORD ENGLISH DICTIONARY.

Most physicians formerly kept their case notes in Latin. An interesting excerpt from the medical records of William Heberden, the English physician after whom the digital osteophytes of degenerative joint disease are named, was published in the *Journal of the American Medical Association* a few years ago. Heberden's COMMENTARIES ON THE HISTORY AND CURE OF DISEASE (published in English in 1802, the year after his death) were based upon a lifetime accumulation of medical records. The records themselves, which are still stored (in Latin manuscript) in the Library of the Royal College of Physicians in London, include notes on the case of Samuel Johnson the lexicographer (5).

The language of primitive pathology is of far less use today than that of medieval anatomy. Whereas anatomy is a descriptive science, pathology inquires into the causes and effects of abnormal processes and states, and before the era of the microscope and of modern analytical chemistry it was, like physiology, a composite of empiricism and superstition, with generous doses of alchemy and wishful thinking.

Some pathological terms that are purely descriptive are as useful today as ever. *Abscessus=a withdrawal or separation* aptly characterizes a soft-tissue infection that is "walled off" from surrounding structures. In this sense it appears in the medical works of the Roman encyclopedist Celsus, who wrote during the lifetime of Christ. Celsus also uses the Latin *cancer=crab* to indicate an eroding and ulcerating lesion. This word has an interesting progeny in the language of modern medicine. We employ it unchanged as an English term for malignancies in general, though with the advance of microscopic pathology it has become more of a lay term than a technical one (6). Even before the Normans carried French into England, the Anglo-Saxons had adopted the Latin

5. McHenry LC: Medical Case Notes on Samuel Johnson in the Heberden Manuscripts. JAMA 195:89, 1966. Johnson buffs, the only readers who will follow up this reference, are warned that the article contains a mistranslation. Heberden was called in to see Johnson on the morning after his stroke, June 17, 1783. Boswell's detailed and poignant description of that event in THE LIFE OF SAMUEL JOHNSON, LL. D. makes it clear that from first to last Johnson's only symptom was aphasia. Heberden's clinical note, based evidently on his illustrious patient's history and his own findings, states *"vox subito perit in viro nato LXXIV, mente et membris illasis; quae intra paucos dies fere restituitur"* ("Sudden loss of speech in a 74-year-old male. No impairment of limbs or mental faculties. Virtually complete recovery within a few days.") The translation offered in the article incorrectly renders the second sentence "Mind and limbs affected."

6. In German, *Krebs=crab* is the usual term employed by laity and physicians alike in speaking of malignant disease. The expression *Krebsmilch,* meaning a white secretion from the nipple in patients with carcinoma of the breast, thus has the somewhat fanciful alternate meaning *crab milk. Carcinoma* is derived from the Greek word for *crab, karkinos.*

term in roughly the same sense as that in which Celsus used it, and the word has come down to us in two corrupt forms: the outmoded *cancrum oris*=*an erosive lesion of the mouth* and the more viable *canker*. This latter word is often used figuratively for a distressing mental preoccupation, and also appears in the lay term *canker sore* for what the physician calls an *aphthous ulcer*. (This makes the physician feel superior and may even in some measure bolster his self-esteem in spite of his awareness that he knows no better than the patient what the lesion is or how to make it go away.) Finally, *chancre*, the French version of *cancer*, has in the past century acquired the specific meaning of the primary ulcer of syphilis.

Lupus=*wolf* had, as early as the tenth century, the figurative meaning of *an erosive ulcer*. *Ranula* is Latin for *a little frog*. *Tinea* means *a worm* (compare the English misnomer *ringworm*) and may originally have been applied to skin diseases caused by tissue nematodes. *Rodent* ulcer recalls the literal meaning of our generic term for rats, mice and other *gnawing* animals. *Furunculus* means *a little thief*. *Fistula* originally signified *tube, pipe* or *reed*, but its application to a sinus tract had already occurred in pre-Christian times.

Angina comes from an Aryan root meaning *compression* or *squeezing*, which has given us, by various routes, *anguish, anxiety* and *anger*. In classic Latin *angina* meant a swelling of the throat, a sense that we preserve in *Ludwig's angina*. Our *angina pectoris*, which restores the ancient idea of squeezing, first appears in the medical literature of the seventeenth century.

Lumbago, from *lumbus*=*loin*, was used in medical Latin as early as the fourth century. A *tophus* is a soft concretion formed in the tissues of persons with gout, and in classic Latin *tofus* meant any soft stone, whence the modern term *tufa* for the volcanic rock around Rome in which the early Christians dug the catacombs. *Delirium* originated in an agricultural metaphor. The verb *delirare*, from *de*=*away* and *lira*=*furrow*, meant *to plow in a crooked line* and was applied figuratively to those who acted irresponsibly or performed senseless actions. The derivation of *claudication* from *claudicare*=*to limp* is curiously belied in such statements as this from a recent journal article: "Since intermittent claudication in the arm occurs only with work and is relieved by rest, it may be misinterpreted as angina pectoris."

When Ambroise Paré developed effective techniques for control of hemorrhage and thus opened the era of modern surgery, the operator was already equipped with a formidable array of instruments, whose design had changed little since the second or third century A.D. The profession of medicine did not in ancient times concern itself with anything remotely resembling surgery; hence the passage in the Oath of Hippocrates, "I will not perform lithotomy, but will not interfere with those who do." The lancing of boils, the suturing of wounds and the extraction of calculi and foreign bodies, as well as operative dentistry, were the province of the so-called barber-surgeons. Unlettered and often itinerant, these practitioners probably did more good in their way than the erudite and cultivated but woefully ineffectual physicians, who chattered learnedly about peccant humors and restorative purges but often declined even to touch their patients.

Modern surgery has borrowed the names for a great many of its instruments directly from classic Latin. The *scalpellum* (or *scalpellus*) is mentioned by Cicero as a surgical knife; the word is a diminutive of *scalprum = cutting tool*. Our modern *vulsellum* appears in classic Latin as *volsella*, meaning *a pair of tweezers*. *Tenaculum* (from *tenere = to hold*) first occurs in English medical writing in the seventeenth century, where it means a forceps with hooked jaws for picking up severed vessels in order to ligate them. *Forceps* itself is Augustan Latin for *tongs* or *pincers*.

In classic Latin *speculum* meant *mirror*, but by the sixteenth century it had acquired a meaning much like its present one, *dilator of orifices*. Since it comes from *specere = to look at*, it may have been coined for this latter application independently of its other meaning. However, before the invention of the electric lamp, an instrument for examining an orifice or cavity had to use reflected light, and was therefore generally equipped with a small plane or concave *mirror*.

Probe comes directly from *proba*, which is good medieval Latin for an instrument used to explore wounds; ultimately it goes back to *probare = to try or prove*. From *temptare* (which means nearly the same thing), by way of French *tenter*, came the Shakespearean synonym for probe, *tent*. (Hamlet: "I'll tent him to the quick.") The *spica* bandage was so named because its alternating oblique folds look like the blades of *an ear of grain*.

When the Swedish naturalist Karl von Linné published his system for the methodic naming of plants and animals in 1735, he based it entirely on Latin. (He also Latinized his own name to Linnaeus.) His system, still in use today in almost the identical form in which he gave it to the world, has been extended to include all new discoveries in the field of natural history, not least important of which have been those made with the microscope. Though the majority of taxonomic terms that have been devised for microorganisms are either eponymous or of Greek origin, a few are pure Latin. For example, a genus of coccal saprophyte that tends to form cubical clusters of eight cells is called *Sarcina* from the fancied resemblance between these clusters and *a soldier's pack*.

Besides taxonomic terms, microbiologists and immunologists use a number of technical words derived from classic Latin: *bacillus* = *a little rod; virus* = *a rank substance, a poison; serum* = *whey*. The last-mentioned term had an ill-defined anatomic significance even in the days of Pliny the Elder, and during the prevalence of the humoral theory *serum* was considered one of the secondary or lesser humors. *Vaccine,* now a general term for any antigenic substance containing pathogenic micro-organisms in an attenuated or inert state, was formerly applied to the infectious material of *vaccinia* (cow-pox), from Latin *vacca* = *cow. Inoculation* is not derived from *inoculum;* quite the reverse. The former word, which is in Shakespeare, used to refer to the engrafting of one plant on another; the latter is a twentieth-century back-formation.

The microscope also extended the horizons of descriptive anatomy and of pathology, so that hundreds of new terms were required. Most of these were taken bodily from Latin *(cilium* = *eyelash; nucleus* = *kernel)* or fashioned out of Latin or Latinized Greek stems *(stratum germinativum, lymphocyte). Lumen* = *light,* referring to the cavity of a hollow or tubular organ, was apparently not used until late in the nineteenth century. The word was probably first employed by microscopists examining cross-sections of vessels, since the empty interior was represented on the slide as a clear area. (Carpenters refer to panes in a sash window as *lights.*)

The new microscopic pathology revolutionized medicine and had some important effects on its terminology. *Tuberculosis* replaced both the physician's expression *phthisis* (Greek, *a wasting away*) and the vernacular *consumption.*

The terms *tubercular* and *tuberculous* are often confounded by physicians as well as by patients. *Tubercular* is a morphologic term applied to a structure *that has tubercles; tuberculous,* formerly synonymous with it, now properly means *pertaining to tuberculosis. Tuberculotic,* once seriously proposed as an alternative to *tuberculous* to eliminate confusion, has been allowed to die quietly. *Scrofula,* a now obsolete term for tuberculous lymphadenitis, comes from *scrofa* = *a brood sow;* apparently the lumpy neck of a patient with this condition reminded people in an agrarian society of the belly of a lactating sow.

Richard von Krafft-Ebing's monumental and controversial study of sexual deviation, PSYCHOPATHIA SEXUALIS, first published in 1886, was written in German except for the most offensive details, which were given in Latin, apparently to prevent their being read by women and others lacking an academic background. The Latin passages were generally preserved in translations into other languages, and it was not until 1965 that a completely English version was published.

A few Latin phrases survive in modern medical parlance from the days when Latin was still known to virtually all educated persons: *curriculum vitae, in situ, in vitro, in vivo, locum tenens.* Latin continues to be the favored medium for the naming of skin diseases, including such typesetter's nightmares as *lichen sclerosus et atrophicus, erythema annulare centrifugum, angiokeratoma corporis diffusum, keratosis pilaris rubra faciei,* and *ectodermosis erosiva pluriorificialis.*

Greek

Cassius: Did Cicero say anything?
Casca: Ay, he spoke Greek.
Cassius: To what effect?
Casca: Nay . . . those that understood him smil'd at one another, and shook their heads; but for mine own part, it was Greek to me.

William Shakespeare
Julius Caesar

The language in which, nearly thirty centuries ago, the blind bard Homer composed his epic poems, the ILIAD and the ODYSSEY, descended from the same Aryan parent tongue as Latin, and the two languages have many roots in common. Moreover, as we have mentioned, the Latins borrowed their alphabet from the Greeks (who had in turn borrowed it from the Phoenicians, who got it from the Egyptians) and adapted it to their own needs.

These are not the only points at which the two languages touch. The Greek civilization was a more advanced one than the Roman; at the time when Rome's chief but all-important claim to distinction was an invincible army, Greece was far ahead in philosophy and belles-lettres, and also in many of the practical sciences, including medicine. When Rome conquered Greece, it absorbed all the best of Greek learning and culture. Greek became the second language of the educated and the leisured class, and served as the official language of the eastern half of the Empire (later known as the Byzantine Empire), corresponding to modern Turkey, the Levant and the Balkans.

Greek words and phrases abounded in Latin writings, and the celebrated MEDITATIONS of the Emperor Marcus Aurelius Antoninus were composed entirely in Greek. As Rome took possession of the arts and sciences of Greece, she borrowed their terminologies also, reshaping many words into Latin. This process of assimilation, which began before the Christian era, accounts for many likenesses between Latin and Greek words that are not due to the common origin of the two languages.

It is scarcely an exaggeration to say that Rome had no practitioners of medicine until after the conquest of Greece. The teachings of Hippocrates were lawful booty along with all other things Greek; indeed, much of the Greek learning, particularly in medicine and astronomy, had originally been filched from the Egyptians after the conquests of Alexander the Great. In the second century A.D. Galen, a brilliant physician of Greek birth and training, settled in Rome and made many important discoveries in anatomy and physiology. In his extensive writings he brought together in encyclopedic fashion all the medical knowledge of his time. It is an astonishing instance of the intellectual and scientific inertia of the Dark Ages that Galen's collected medical works (of which about one hundred survive to this day) were regarded as the universal and unquestionable authority in medicine for no fewer than fourteen centuries. This fact is all the more staggering when we consider that a modern medical treatise may become dangerously obsolete within three or four years.

It was chiefly in Latin and Arabic translations that Galen's works were handed down through the ages, for the language and literature of ancient Greece had a very different fate than those of Rome. Whereas the Latin language was kept alive down through the centuries by the Christian Church, no such institution existed to maintain a widespread knowledge of Greek once the Byzantine Empire began to shrink and disintegrate. Even though the New Testament (except for St. Matthew's Gospel) was written originally in Greek, it was in the Latin Vulgate edition that it was used by the early Christians as a medium of proselytism, instruction and worship.

The rediscovery of the Greek cultural and literary heritage in the Renaissance was much delayed by these circumstances. Though the Greek language has evolved no more in twenty-five centuries than has English in five, so that a modern Greek can read Homer in the classical version without great difficulty, few of the most learned scholars in western Europe were able to do so between the sixth and the sixteenth centuries. The works of Aristotle were all but lost to the western world until the disciples of the Arabic philosophers Avicenna and Averroes entered into communication with the adherents of Scholasticism in the eleventh and twelfth centuries. The Latin versions of Aristotle that appeared then in western Europe were not direct translations from the original Greek. These writings had passed through Syrian, Arabic, and sometimes Hebrew before arriving in a language that western scholars could understand.

By the time the full tide of the Renaissance reached England, around the time of Henry VIII, Latin was firmly established there as the language of scholarship and the medium of college-level instruction. Greek, on the other hand, was all but unknown, and the efforts of a few scholars to introduce the study of the Greek language and literature into the university curriculum met with vigorous opposition from the majority. In allusion to the ten years' war recorded in the ILIAD, the opponents of the "Greeks" were styled "Trojans."

But by the seventeenth century Greek occupied a position second only to Latin as a classical study. Though few scholars attained great proficiency in speaking it (as many did in Latin), it was taken for granted by polite writers that every educated man knew enough Greek to decipher words coined from that language.

Almost from its origin, the English tongue had been receiving a slow but steady accession of words from Greek, often through Latin. *Asbestos, chaos, character, dogma, echo, emphasis, horizon* and *idea* are pure Greek. Several medical terms that look like venerable English natives are in fact of Greek origin. *Dropsy* and *palsy* are corruptions of *hydrops* and *paralysis,* and both probably found their way into everyday English by way of Bible translations (Luke 14:2; Mark 2:3). *Pleurisy* is a corruption of *pleuritis, rickets* of *rachitis.*

Quinsy, too, is ultimately Greek, and has a colorful origin. The Latin term for a severe sore throat was *quinancia* (or *squinancia*), and it is from this word that *quinsy* passed directly into English, probably before the fifteenth century. The Latin expression was in turn derived from Greek *kynanche=a dog collar* or *choke-halter (kyon=dog* and *anche =choking),* a vivid evocation of the plight of the unfortunate patient with a peritonsillar abscess.

Most technical terms derived from Greek have preserved more of the original spelling and pronunciation than these examples, and for that reason they tend to give English-speaking persons a lot more trouble than do terms derived from Latin. To understand this, we must consider, first, that though Greek is an Aryan language like both Latin and English, it is more "Oriental" than either of them, and more akin phonetically to Russian or Hindustani than to the Romance and Teutonic languages spoken throughout most of the western world.

Secondly, though the Greek alphabet was the ancestor of our own, the two are sufficiently different that our spelling of words derived from Greek is only an approximation to the correct Greek orthography. For example, the sounds *ps* and *th* are each expressed by a single letter in

Greek. The relatively common combinations *ng* and *nx* in English terms of Greek origin *(angioma, pharynx)* were spelled *gg* and *gx* by the Greeks: *aggeion=vessel, pharygx=throat.*

Most Greek stems have come into English by way of Latin, and we are indebted to the Romans for many of the conventions used in transliterating them. The Romans Latinized the inflectional endings of most Greek words, though a few, like *colon, hypospadias, opisthotonos* and *systole,* have retained their original terminations.

The Greek alphabet had no *c* and the Roman had no *k;* hence, a Roman *c* was often used as the equivalent of Greek *k.* When this substutited *c* precedes *e, i* or *y* in modern English words *(cephalic, cirrhosis, cycle)* it is given a soft or sibilant sound instead of the historically correct *k* sound. We occasionally find the *k* preserved before *e, i* or *y (kerion, kymograph),* and in the case of a few roots both *c* and *k* forms exist side by side: *cerumen–keratin, cinematograph–kinase.* Oddly, in *keloid* and in the prefix *kilo– (thousand)* the *k* represents Greek *chi,* ordinarily rendered by *ch* as in *cheilosis, choledochus.*

In other modern languages there is no more uniformity; compare French *kyste, cycle* and Spanish *quiste, ciclo.* German often renders the softened *k* by initial *z: Zyste, Zyklus;* but contrast *Kinetik.* Despite these examples, the modern Teutonic languages other than English have made but sparing use of Latin and Greek material. Most Latin roots in German popular speech have come in through modern French *(Differenz, interessant, Motif)* or are survivals from academic Latin: *Datum= date of the month, Rektor, prosit* (drinking toast). Modern scientific German makes extensive use of native Teutonic roots. For instance, the German for *lingual papillae* is *Zungenwärzchen* ("little tongue-warts"); for *tenosynovitis, Sehnenscheidenentzündung* ("sinew-sheath enkindling") and for *mucous membrane, Schleimhaut* ("slime-skin"). German also readily forms compounds between classic and Teutonic language materials, as in *Kernikterus,* from German *Kern=nut, basal ganglion* and Greek *ikteros=jaundice.* In a few instances this German practice has influenced coinage of English technical words. German *Antikörper* was undoubtedly the model for the rare Greek–English hybrid *antibody.* (Others are *bioavailability* and *sicklemia.*)

Pairings of consonants that seem to us to be practically unpronounceable are characteristic of Greek. When such a pair occurs at the beginning of a word (as in *bdellium, cnidophore, ctenophore, mnemonic, pneumonia, ptyalin, psittacosis* [7]), we suppress the first consonant. Only

7. The presence of any of these consonant pairs, of *ch* or *th,* or of *y* used as a vowel, generally indicates that a term is of Greek origin. This is not always true, however. In

when a vowel precedes the pair *(gastrocnemius, amnesia, hypercapnea)* do we pronounce both consonants. In *diphtheria, naphthalene* and *ophthalmic* the *ph* is often incorrectly pronounced like *p,* while in *dyspnea* the *p* is sometimes practically inaudible. The *th* in *asthma* is no longer sounded at all, but like the now-silent *p* in *raspberry* it confers on the preceding *s* the sound of *z.*

The Greeks had no letter corresponding to our *h,* but they signified a harsh breathing at the beginning of certain words by a sort of diacritical mark like a backwards apostrophe. Words beginning with *r* were invariably adorned with this mark, whence we get such forms as *rhinitis* and *rhodopsin,* in which the unpronounced *h* has not only been needlessly retained but has been shifted to the other side of the *r.* When this combination follows a vowel within a word, the spelling is further complicated by the addition of an entirely superfluous second *r: diarrhea, scirrhous, cardiorrhexis.*

Although prefixes such as *cata–* and *epi–* retain their final vowels before full-fledged consonants *(catalepsy, epidemic),* they shed them before the rough breathing. Moreover, their own terminal consonants then blend phonetically with the Greek *"h": cathode, ephedrine.* (Contrast English compounds like *sweetheart* and *haphazard* in which the *h* sound is kept distinct.) The modern practice is to ignore the rough breathing in the stem *hem–* (from *haime=blood*) unless it occurs at the beginning of a word. Thus, though we write *hematology,* we do not write *hypophosphathemia* or *hyperliphemia. Leukemia* is a corruption of the more correct *leuchaemia* originally proposed by Virchow.

The Greeks' fondness for stringing together several vowels and diphthongs in a row made their language musical to the ear but introduced many letters that we deem superfluous. Greek *ai* and *oi* usually appear in modern American English as *e (hemorrhage, celiac),* though the variant spellings with *ae* and *oe (haemorrhage, coeliac)* are favored in Canada and Great Britain. The British spelling is occasionally of use in distinguishing two similar stems, as in the case of *ped–,* from Latin *pes =foot,* and *paed–,* from Greek *pais=child.* Both appear as *ped–* in American spelling, hence the antidiluvian joke about the man who took his foot trouble to a pediatrician. An awareness of the alternate spelling is necessary in looking up words like *aetiology* and *oesophagus* in the index of a British work.

A simple *i* is usually substituted for Greek *ei (Phthirus, chiropody)*

---

tophus, ph has been erroneously substituted for Latin *f.* On the other hand, the modern spelling *lacrimal* conceals the Greek origin of the word, which would more correctly be rendered *lachrymal.*

though sometimes it is the *e* that survives *(trachea)*. The Greek letter *upsilon* usually turns into *y* in English *(hyphema, chyle)* unless it follows another vowel. After *a* or *e* we render it as a *u (trauma, neuron)* and when it is preceded by *o*, with rare exceptions like *acoustic*, we drop the *o* and write simply *u (urine)*.

Spanish and Italian, however, drop the *u* and keep the *o: orina*. The transliteration of Greek words into the Roman alphabet is by no means uniform among Romance languages. Spanish, Portuguese, and Italian consistently change *ph* to f *(farmacia)*, ch to c *(tecnica)* and th to t *(ortopedia)*. All three render Greek *upsilon* as *i (citoplasma)*, and Italian invariably omits the *h* with which other languages indicate the Greek rough breathing *(emorragia)* and renders *x* (the Greek letter *xi*) by *ss: ossigeno*. In Romance languages other than French, Greek *m* is changed to *n* before the *f (ph)* sound: *enfisema, linfonodo*. This shift from *m* to *n* for the sake of euphony is indeed curious, for the Greek notion of euphony demanded precisely the opposite change before *ph:* the first syllable of *emphysema* is a phonetic variant of the preposition *en*. French transliterates Greek words in much the same way as English, but changes *–ia* to *–ie (anémie)*, *–itis* to *–ite (appendicite)* and *–osis* to *–ose (tuberculose)*. Compare Italian *anemia, appendicite, tuberculosi*.

In *eschar* and *schizophrenia*, speakers of English almost invariably give the *ch* its correct Greek sound of *k*, but in certain other words of Greek origin *(ischium, schistosomiasis)* the combination *sch* is often erroneously pronounced *sh*, probably because of the example of terms and names borrowed from German *(Weltanschauung, Schick)*.

Another sort of confusion arises in the case of words derived from Greek and containing *–ng–* preceded and followed by vowels. English has three ways of pronouncing the *ng* combination, as exemplified in *danger, anger* and *hanger*. The *nj* sound, as in the first example, is found chiefly in words from Greek or Latin *(angel, vengeance, arranged)* and in words in which the *n* and the vowel preceding it constitute a prefix, or part of one *(congestion, ungentlemanly)*.

The hard *g* sound occurs most often in words derived from Anglo-Saxon roots: *hunger, finger, linger*, while the liquid *ng* is characteristic of derived forms in which the following vowel is part of a suffix *(singer, longing, hangover)*.

Despite the intricacy of this pattern of variations, English has one inviolable rule regarding the *ng* combination: when followed by *a, o* or *u*, the *g* in this combination is never given a *j* sound. Though the average speaker has no difficulty in following this rule with everyday words like *hangar, bungalow, ingot, tango, lingual* and *fungus*, the rule is violated often in such medical terms as *meningocele* and *laryngospasm*.

The source of this kind of mispronunciation is obvious. Words derived from the stems *mening–* and *laryng–* in which the *j* sound is correct *(meningitis, laryngeal)* are more commonly used than are the forms in which the *ng* is followed by *o*. The erroneous pronunciation *meninjocele*, then, reflects the operation of a speech habit beyond its proper sphere. In the case of *–ng–* stems not usually followed by *o* or *i* we seldom hear an incorrect *j* sound before *o: sphingomyelin, myringotomy.*

The double *o* in Greek words is yet another source of difficulty. Unlike English and Dutch, in which this combination is a diphthong, Greek does not combine the two *o*'s of *oon=egg* or *zoon=animal* in a single sound. These two *o*'s are actually two different letters in Greek; the first is *omega* or long *o*, the second *omicron* or short *o*. The fact that they ought to be pronounced separately is sometimes indicated by placing a diaeresis over the second *o*, as was formerly done with English words like *coöperate* and *coördinate*. Though in the first syllables of *oöcyst* and *zoölogy* the distinction is usually observed, *oöphorectomy* is quite generally pronounced *ooforectomy*. (A colleague has suggested that the proper pronunciation has fallen into disuse because "oh! oh!" is an expression that must never be heard in the operating room. I reject this explanation on the grounds that "oof!" is equally taboo there.)

Many of the terms of modern anatomy are ultimately Greek in origin, though most have gone through the Latinization process. The Greek anatomic terms are often as colorfully figurative as the Latin ones, though fewer in number. *Pylorus*, for example, means *gatekeeper*. The *tragus* of the ear is so called because in later life it develops a tuft of hair similar in appearance to the beard of a *goat*. The *mitral* valve is shaped like a bishop's *mitre* (from Greek *mitra*). The *carotid* artery gets its name from the fact that pressure upon it can induce unconsciousness *(karoun=to stupefy).*

Many Greek anatomic terms end in *–oid*, from *eidos=form, shape, appearance*. *Ethmoid* and *thyroid* mean respectively *sieve-like* and *shield-like*. *Deltoid, hyoid, lambdoid* and *sigmoid* are allusions to the shapes of Greek letters.

Our *disk* is directly from Greek *diskos*, the round flat stone hurled by the *diskeutes* in athletic contests. (We use other derivatives of the same root when we speak of a Petri *dish*, a chart *desk*, or a speakers' *daïs*.) The *azygos* vein is so designated because it is *without a twin* on the left side of the chest. *Collagen* comes from *kolla=glue.*

The *hemorrhoidal* vessels are among the few structures in the body named from a disease state to which they are subject. The primitive term, *hemorrhoides* (from *haime=blood* and *rhein=to flow*) was applied to bleeding piles, and only afterwards, by extension, to the same vessels in their normal state. A similar history is attached to *ganglion*. The pathological meaning, *a bland swelling on or near a tendon,* was the original one; it was Galen who first employed the term in its modern anatomical significance of a normal thickening along the course of a nerve.

Several medical terms have come down to us from the root embodied in *phlegein=to burn.* *Phlegmon* originally meant *a fire,* and was later extended to *inflammation,* a significance preserved in *phlegmonous gastritis.* *Phlegm* (now strictly a lay term) was early applied to the nasopharyngeal secretion, one of the four humors of primitive physiology, which was thought to be produced by the "combustion" of ingested food. *Phlox=flame* is the name of a brilliant red flower and *phloxine* is a red stain used in histology. *Phlogiston=something burnt* was Lavoisier's designation for the component of air that is consumed by burning; Priestley later substituted *oxygen (oxys=acid* and *genes=forming)* on the analogy of Lavoisier's own *hydrogen.* The stem *phlogist–* has been revived in modern times in the adjective *antiphlogistic,* which is applied to drugs that suppress inflammation.

Anthrax=a hot coal (compare modern *anthracite*) was applied metaphorically to *a boil* in ancient times, but more recently has become the name of a specific infectious disease whose first stage is signalized by the appearance of a solitary sore (8). Whether the name of another such disease, syphilis, is also derived from Greek is open to question. In 1530 the Veronese physician Girolamo Fracastoro published a Latin poem, *Syphilis, sive Morbus Gallicus (Syphilis, or the French Disease),* containing a fanciful account of the origin of the disease. Fracastoro's term was adapted from the name of his hero, Syphilus. As his more serious writings make plain, he was as uncertain as his contemporaries about the venereal transmission of the disease; in his poem it is a punishment for impiety, not fornication. Hence there is no basis for the derivation of Syphilus from *syn=with* and *philos=love.* The theory that the first syllable represents Greek *sys=pig* is equally implausible, for Syphilus was a shepherd, not a swineherd.

The Greek *typhos* means *smoke.* This word was assumed into Late Latin as *typhus* with the meaning of *pride or arrogance* but later died out in this sense, only to be resurrected in the eighteenth century as the name of a disease that causes, among other symptoms, a clouding of the mental faculties. *Erysipelas* was known to Hippocrates; the derivation

---

8. *Anthracosis* signified, in classic Greek, a malignant ulcer; the modern meaning of the term is derived from the literal sense of *anthrax.* The Latin *carbunculus,* in ancient times synonymous with *anthrax,* also means *a coal.*

of the word is probably from *erysis*=*redness* and *pella*=*skin,* though THE OXFORD ENGLISH DICTIONARY is skeptical of this etymology. *Diabetes* is from *diabainein*=*to flow through,* and *exanthem* from *exanthein*=*to blossom forth. Nausea* (Greek *nausia*), from the same root as *nautical* and *navigation,* at first meant strictly *seasickness.*

In classic Greek the ending *–itis* was an adjectival suffix like English *–ous* or *–ish,* to be stuck on the end of a noun. Thus, from *arthron* =*joint* could be fashioned the adjective *arthritis*=*of or pertaining to a joint or joints.* The phrase *nosos arthritis* (9), then, meant *a disease of joints.* In time the noun was omitted, and the adjective remained to carry on the work alone. By convention, *–itis* now has a restricted meaning, *inflammation of.* Until comparatively recently this suffix was pronounced *eetis* in English.

A similar tale hangs by the ending *–osis,* which was originally used to form nouns from verbs, as in the case of *amaurosis,* from *amaurein* =*to darken.* Later the ending came to be tacked on to adjectives (*cyanosis,* from *cyan*=*blue*), nouns (*thrombosis,* from *thrombos*=*lump*) and even words of Latin origin (*pediculosis,* from Latin *pediculus*=*little foot,* a reference to the shape of the body louse). It now has the general connotation of *an abnormal state or condition,* as in *keratosis, mucoviscidosis, psychoneurosis,* though in many older words (*anastomosis, aponeurosis, diagnosis*) this significance is not present. The idea of *an excess of some normal substance, tissue or cell* may be expressed by the joint use of *hyper–* and *–osis,* as in *hyperhidrosis,* but more often such words dispense with the prefix: *hemochromatosis, gliosis, lymphocytosis.* Finally, *–osis* can denote *the presence of a foreign and usually noxious substance: asbestosis, bagassosis.*

From the Greek word for *bow, toxon* (compare *toxophily*=*archery*), is derived the term *toxic,* whence *toxicology, toxigenic* and *antitoxin.* The adjective *toxikos,* originally meaning *of or pertaining to archery,* later acquired a narrower significance, referring solely to poisonous substances in which arrows were dipped. *Tetanus* (*tetanos*)=*muscular spasm* was applied specifically to lockjaw even in Hippocrates' day. *Tetany* is a much more modern term derived from the same origin by way of French *tétanie.* From *kline*=*bed* came the ancient Greek word *klinikos* for a physician who visits his patients while they are confined by illness, and *klinike,* the art or method of such a physician. *Chronic* is from

9. It should be noted that *–itis* is a feminine ending, agreeing in gender with *nosos* =*disease.* For this reason medical nouns ending in *–itis* are feminine, and any qualifying Latin adjectives must also be feminine: *linitis plastica, retinitis pigmentosa.* The corresponding masculine adjective ending, *–ites,* is without issue in modern technical terminology; the nouns *ascites* and *tympanites* are formed on a different principle.

chronos=time, and was used in its modern sense, and contrasted with *acute,* as early as the fifth century by the Numidian medical writer Caelius Aurelianus. *Acute* (Latin *acutus=sharp*) was applied to illnesses of rapid course and short duration even earlier, and appears in Celsus.

Our somewhat derogatory epithet *hypochondriac* began life as an anatomic term meaning *under the [costal] cartilages.* In humoral pathophysiology the right and left hypochondria were considered the seats of a wide variety of constitutional disorders because they housed the liver and the spleen. Imaginary and psychosomatic illnesses were formerly blamed largely on these organs, whence the expressions (now nearly obsolete) *liverish, bilious* and *splenetic. Hypochondriasis* seems to be a relatively modern coinage referring to the state of mind of one whom the layperson calls a *hypochondriac* (for whom the physician has his own set of more explicit and less kindly terms).

Diathesis at first meant simply *a state or condition.* Later it was applied to certain abnormal constitutional states, as in *hemorrhagic diathesis;* now it can denote *any abnormal state. Hectic,* originally meaning *habitual or constitutional,* was later restricted to febrile illnesses, but with the advance of differential diagnosis it has been abandoned by the physician and appropriated by the citizenry at large.

A number of medical terms of Greek origin that were once common in both professional and vernacular use have virtually dropped out of the language, including *apoplexy, clyster* (also spelled *glister*) and *hydrophobia,* for which we have substituted *stroke, enema* and *rabies. Catarrh (katarrhous=a flowing down)* was formerly overworked, for it could connote anything from the common cold to diarrhea ("intestinal catarrh") or hepatitis ("catarrhal jaundice"). But it was a useful word for all that, and a more compact and euphonious expression than *postnasal drip.* We still speak of the *catarrhal* stages of measles and whooping cough.

Another pathologic term from Greek that has died out is *imposthume.* The original Greek form was *apostema,* which, like Latin *abscessus,* means *cut off, withdrawn.* The French corrupted the word to *empostume* (though Rabelais spells it *aposteme*), and the English further corrupted it to *imposthume.* The insertion of an *h* into this word is analogous to the process by which English has turned *postumus* (Latin for *last*) into *posthumous.* Apparently the Latin word was erroneously traced to *post =after* and *humus=the ground,* or, figuratively, *the grave.* Many English words contain letters inserted by well-intentioned nincompoops with a smattering of some classical or modern language who either arrived at false conclusions regarding the sources of words or sought to rectify "corrupt" spellings. The *h* in *rhyme* and the *s* in *aisle* and *island* are examples of the first, the *b* in *doubt* and the *c* in *scissors* and *scythe* are examples of the second.

In Middle English the science of medicine was called *physick,* from the Greek word referring to the material world. Though this term survived into the nineteenth century, it has now largely fallen out of use, partly in deference to its brother *physics.* It survives only in the derivative *physician* and in the lay term for a laxative, *physic.*

It happens occasionally in most languages that words of entirely different origin come to be regarded as related in meaning because they are similar in form. English is full of unrelated look-alikes: *admiral* is not derived from *admire,* nor *belfry* from *bell,* nor *cutlet* from *cut.* Similarly, in medical terminology two words of quite distinct derivation sometimes bear a striking resemblance to one another: *anorectal–anorectic, semicoma–seminoma, septal–septic.* On the other hand, many word pairs that are genuine cognates have widely divergent meanings: *deduce–deduct, ileum–ilium, glaucous–glaucoma.* Is it any wonder that the student of pathology has difficulty in distinguishing *granulation, granuloma, granulocyte* and *granulosa cell tumor?*

Though the tracing of word origins is, in general, merely an amusing pastime, it does help to distinguish between words whose family resemblance is illusory. Medical terms of Greek origin seem particularly liable to this kind of confusion.

The Greek *eschara* meant variously *hearth, camp fire* and *pan of coals.* By metaphorical extension it had acquired even in Hippocrates' time the meaning of *the scab that forms on a burn.* It has come down to us in the modern terms *eschar, escharotic* and *scar;* but *scarify* is from *skariphos* =*stylus.*

Basilic is derived from the Greek word for *royal,* but *basilar,* like *base* and *basal,* comes from a different word meaning *pedestal.* *Canthus (kanthos),* which meant to the ancient Greeks just what it means to us today, has no connection with *acanthosis* (from *akantha* =*thorn, thistle*).

Myocardium contains the stem *my–* (from *mys*=*mouse, muscle*), but *mylohyoid* gets its first syllable from *myle*=*mill, molar tooth,* and *myelitis* gets its from still a third word, *myelos*=*marrow.* There exists in medical terminology an exactly analogous set of stems beginning with *p: pyoderma,* from *pyon*=*pus; pylephlebitis,* from *pyle*=*gate;* and *pyelitis,* from *pyelos*=*pelvis.*

The need to manufacture new terms to keep pace with the progress of scientific medicine occasionally results in an overworking of the mine. Now and then the process comes up with a "new" word that already means something else. *Dermatome,* coined from two Greek words meaning *skin* and *cut*, is a perfectly satisfactory term for a surgical instrument designed to cut skin in preparation for grafting. But besides that meaning, it has an entirely different one: a zone of the skin surface supplied by sensory branches of a single spinal cord segment. *Scaphoid* = *boat-like* is the name of two different bones, one in the wrist and the other in the ankle, both of which are more frequently called *navicular*, from the Latin for *little boat*. We also speak of a *scaphoid* abdomen by a simile of very different purport.

Dyscrasia appears in the writings of Plutarch with the nebulous meaning of *a bad temperament of the air*. In modern medicine it has two other meanings, one of them equally nebulous: a *food dyscrasia* is a dislike or intolerance for certain kinds of food, and a *blood dyscrasia* means something wrong with the production of the cellular elements of the blood.

The Greek stem *path*– forms two entirely different classes of English words. In *pathology, adenopathy, idiopathic* and *psychopath* it preserves its original meaning *(pathos = suffering)*, but in *naturopathy, homeopathic* and *osteopath* it refers to *treatment*. The stem *gen*– (from *gennan* = *to beget*) has likewise begotten two distinct lines of offspring: in *pathogenic, diabetogenic* and *goitrogenic* (10) it means *causative of*, whereas in *cryptogenic, psychogenic* and *cardiogenic* it means *caused by or originating in*. In some words *(e.g., allergenic, mutagenic)* it can have either meaning. The closely allied suffix –*genous* adds another set of alternative meanings: in *hematogenous* it signifies *carried by*, and in *myelogenous* and *nephrogenous* it indicates the place where something is generated or begotten. Of all these adjectival variants only the first meaning of –*genic* has a corresponding series of nouns ending in –*genesis*.

Not to belabor the Greeks unduly, we can cite some anatomical homonyms from Latin that also cause confusion at times. For example, *natal* has two distinct meanings, one from *natus* = *newborn* and the other from *nates* = *buttocks*. *Mental* can refer either to the *mind (mens)* or to the *chin (mentum)*. Latin *os* means both *bone* and *mouth*. At least we can tell the difference in compound words, where the form meaning *bone* becomes *oss*– (not to be confused with *ost*– from Greek *osteon*) and the form meaning *mouth* becomes *or*–.

As Greek and Latin are both descendants of common Aryan, it is not susprising that they display many lexical similarities. Among Latin–

---

10. *Goitre* is old French, from Latin *guttur* = *throat* (compare *guttural*). *Goitrogenic* is one of several compounds of French and Greek in medical terminology; others include *bagassosis, bunionectomy* and *chancroid*. Perhaps the most unconventional is *culdoscopy*, from *cul-de-sac*.

Greek cognate pairs of importance in medical terminology may be mentioned the following nouns: Greek *argyros* and Latin *argentum* = silver; *cardia* and *cor* = heart; *gala* and *lac* = milk; *hyster* and *uterus* = womb; *lykos* and *lupus* = wolf; *mys* and *mus* = mouse; *nyx* and *nox* = night; *odous* and *dens* = tooth; *onyx* and *unguis* = nail; *oon* and *ovum* = egg; *ophthalmos* and *oculus* = eye; *pneumon* and *pulmo* = lung; *pous* and *pes* = foot.

4

a museum in words

If you want to examine a set of cupping glasses or a pill tile, you will have to visit a museum or a private collection of medical curios. If you want to view the pyramids or the Himalayas, you will have to travel. However, a wealth of fascinating materials from other times and places is preserved for us in our very midst, like a fly in amber, in the language we use daily. Many expressions current in English have been borrowed directly from modern foreign languages. Many others are derived from proper names of persons and places. If we define a museum as a collection of curios and artifacts from ancient times and remote places, of works of art and the effects of celebrated persons, surely it takes no great stretch of the imagination to see in language itself a sort of museum.

Technical terminology, like the vernacular, is a rich storehouse of the antique and the exotic. The periodic table of the elements might almost have been conceived as a paradigm of the extremely various sources of technical language. First we have Anglo-Saxon words like *gold, silver* and *lead.* The symbols for these three elements are taken from their international designations, which are Latin: *aurum, argentum* and *plumbum.* Other names formed from Latin stems are *calcium* and *radium,* while *potassium* is a Latinization of English *pot ash.* From Greek stems we have *barium, bromine* and *phosphorus;* from Arabic, *antimony* and *arsenic;* from German, *bismuth* and *zinc. Zirconium* is of Persian origin, *iron* is Celtic and *tungsten* is Swedish.

More than half the elements are named after real or mythical persons or places. There are references to Roman mythology in *mercury* and *titanium;* to Greek mythology in *palladium* and *promethium;* to Norse mythology in *thorium* and *vanadium. Cobalt* and *nickel* are named from superstitions popular in eighteenth-century Europe. *Cadmium, curium* and *gadolinium* are eponyms, while *berkelium, californium* and *americium* are just three of more than twenty elements named after places.

Whereas the kind of word origins we discussed in the previous chapter are after all rather prosaic except to a classicist, we are now going to investigate some etymologies of a more intriguing type. Before we do so, it may be advisable to make one or two general observations about the tracing of word origins.

Though all the etymologies given in this book are supported by reliable philologic authority, they cannot all be urged with equal probability. The scientific tracing of the origins of words demands painstaking research through many languages and literatures, often spanning hundreds of years. Until comparatively modern times etymology was based largely on guesswork; indeed, the origins suggested for some common Latin words by the Roman grammarians Varro, Donatus and Quintilian are nothing short of ridiculous.

Grammarians are not the only ones who go astray in tracing word origins. It would be hard to overestimate the influence exerted by folk etymology on the ceaseless interplay of form and meaning in living languages. *Equerry* is a variant form of *squire,* both from French *écuyer* and ultimately descended from Latin *scutum = shield* (compare *escutcheon*). But speakers of English have been so long accustomed to associating *equerry* with *equestrian* (from Latin *equus = horse*) that the former word has virtually lost its literal meaning and come to mean something else. *Rotisserie,* despite a widespread misconception extending even to manufacturers of rotisseries, has nothing to do with *rotation.* Derived from French *rôtir = to roast,* the word means a cooking apparatus of the Dutch-oven type, with or without a turning spit.

Folk etymology can be a formidable obstacle to the accurate tracing of a root back through time to its "source" in the earliest language of which written records survive. For example, some authorities assert that *borax* is derived from Arabic *baraqa = to glisten,* while others trace it to Persian *burah = white.* Each of these etymologies is based partly on speculation and partly on long-standing tradition, and though neither of them can be proven with unequivocal written evidence, neither can be altogether discounted.

In sharp contrast to *borax, tendon* can be traced back with certainty through a medieval Latin form *tendo* forming oblique cases in *tendon–,* to an earlier Latin *tendo* forming oblique cases in *tendin–,* thence to classic Greek *tenon* forming *tenont–,* derived in its turn from the verb *teinein = to stretch,* which has cognates in virtually all Aryan tongues from Sanskrit onward. As the example of *equerry* and *rotisserie* should make clear, the similarity between modern *tendon* and Greek *tenon* in both form and meaning carries very little weight. On the other hand, the various evolutionary forms of the word appear in the writings of the great classical and medieval anatomists as well as in those of many lesser authorities spanning the years between them. In the face of this copious documentary evidence, no one can seriously question the derivation of *tendon.*

Historical Curiosities

That the English language may be more easily understood, it is necessary to inquire how its derivative words are deduced from their primitives, and how the primitives are borrowed from other languages.

Samuel Johnson
A Grammar of the English Tongue

Analysis of medical terms in current use often indicates that they now mean something quite different than when they were first coined or appropriated by physicians, and often sheds light on the evolution of knowledge about diseases and their treatment.

Errors and misconceptions of former times are embalmed in terms like *cholera,* so called because the diarrhea and vomiting characteristic of the disease were believed to be a discharge of malignant bilious humor *(chole=bile),* and *gonorrhea,* which means literally *a flow of semen.* *Hysteria* is so named because in ancient times the uterus *(hyster)* was considered a seat of mental afflictions. There is another allusion to this notion in *globus hystericus,* which refers to the primitive belief that the "lump in the throat" of a distraught woman was the uterine fundus.

The *pituitary* gland was thought by ancient anatomists to be the source of nasopharyngeal mucus (Latin *pituita=phlegm*), another of the humors. The Greek word for this humor was *rheuma,* from the verb meaning *to flow. Rheum* is now obsolete as an English term for nasal discharge, but the stem survives in *rheumatic fever* and *rheumatoid arthritis.*

From the name of a third humor, *black bile,* come our psychiatric term *melancholia* and the much commoner lay word *melancholy,* often used as an adjective. *Gout* is a very old word borrowed from French and derived ultimately from Latin *gutta=drop* (compare the modern abbreviation *gtt.*). The disease was given this name because deposits of urate crystals were believed to be "drops" of some noxious humor. *Gout* was formerly a slang expression for syphilis; moreover, it is evident that before the biochemical era it was applied to many cases of degenerative and rheumatoid arthritis.

Though there are only a few remnants of humoral pathophysiology in the modern language of medicine, the vernacular retains quite a number of allusions to this old theory; we still hear references to *sanguine, phlegmatic* and *choleric* temperaments, and often speak of being in a good (or bad) *humor.* Little if anything of the astrological side of ancient medicine survives in modern language besides the lay term *lunatic.*

The medieval anatomists spoke of subcutaneous tissue as *areolar = full of small open spaces* because in their inadequately preserved cadavers they generally found this tissue inflated with gases of putrefaction. *Arteries* appeared empty after death and so were believed to be *air passages.* The *jejunum* was also generally found *empty.* Because on gross examination it appeared to be *all flesh,* the digestive gland in the left upper quadrant of the abdomen was called *pancreas.*

Some terms ending in *–oid* bear testimony to early confusion between similar diseases *(typhoid, chancroid),* while others *(sarcoid, keloid)* have no such associations.

The adjective *phrenic,* which in modern use is a synonym for *diaphragmatic,* formerly had a much wider application; Greek *phren* means *mind* as well as *diaphragm* (compare *schizophrenia*). From this significance have come our English words *frenzy* and *frantic,* which were formerly spelled *phrenesy* and *phrenetic.*

𝔅orrowings from 𝔐odern 𝔉oreign 𝔏anguages

I have often wished, that as in our constitution there are several persons whose business it is to watch over our laws, our liberties, and our commerce, certain men might be set apart as superintendants of our language, to hinder any words of a foreign coin from passing among us; and in particular to prohibit any French phrases from becoming current in this kingdom, when those of our own stamp are altogether as valuable.

Joseph Addison
Spectator, No. 165

The patterns according to which words of one language have been borrowed by another often shed light on the relations between two races or nations. In English usage, for example, it is no accident that many words related to music and art are from Italian *(cantata, chiaros-*

curo, solo), many nautical terms are from Dutch *(keel, skipper, sloop)*, and many expressions used in military engineering are from French *(chevaux de frise, redan, salient)*.

Several German words have come into our medical vocabulary through the influence of Virchow, the founder of microscopic pathology, and his disciples: *gitter, mast, stab* and *wasserhelle* cells, *anlage* and *polkissen*. Einthoven's touch persists in the *K* of *EKG (Elektrokardiogramm)*, Gmelin's in the *k* of *ketone (Keton,* a variation on *acetone)*. From Billroth and his school we have *magenstrasze.* from Neufeld the *quellung* reaction. *Mittelschmerz* is a venerable expression for ovulatory pain, and *trichterbrust* and *pfundnase* are old names for anatomic peculiarities. More recent loans include the *blutwelle* of pulmonary embolism and the *spinnbarkeit* of cervical mucus. The *0* and *H* antigens of *Salmonella typhi* are so designated because colonies of flagellated microorganisms (originally, *Proteus vulgaris)* spread over an agar medium in a thin film *(Hauch),* whereas nonflagellated colonies are compact and discrete *(ohne Hauch=without film)*.

French borrowings are even more abundant than German ones in modern medical "English." In clinical medicine we have *bruit, chancre, goitre, grand mal* and *petit mal, grippe, malaise* and *rale;* in surgery, *bougie, curette, débridement, douche, lavage, rongeur* and *tamponade*. The radiologist (who calls a film holder a *cassette)* describes a *niche en plateau* and a *coeur en sabot,* the dermatologist speaks of *café au lait* spots and *formes frustes* (1). The clinical pathologist may use a *burette* to determine a *titre,* and even if he possesses a very powerful *loupe* he will probably need to resort to a microscope to see *organelles* and *rouleaux*. The physical therapist employs *massage* and its more esoteric brethren *effleurage* and *pétrissage*.

Many a patient ends up in the *morgue*. Though this word looks as though it ought to be related to *mort=death,* that is not the case. Used first in France to designate a room where living persons picked up by the police for vagrancy were detained for questioning, *morgue* was only later applied to a repository for the dead. It has been traced with some plausibility to medieval French *morguer=to stare at, to regard sullenly*.

Many French words of even comparatively recent assumption into English have begun an assimilation process. We often encounter such

1. Though often supposed to be from the same source as *frustrate*, the French word *fruste,* which means *battered, worn,* or *defaced,* comes from Latin *frustum=morsel, fragment.* An accurate interpretation of the phrase *forme fruste* is *a variant or atypical form,* not *an undeveloped, abortive or arrested condition*.

usages as *to rongeur* and *ballottable*. French phrases are sometimes partly translated into English, as when *fièvre boutonneuse* becomes *boutonneuse fever* and *spondylite rhizomélique* becomes *rhizomélique spondylitis*. In *iris bombé* the French spelling is preserved but *iris* is given its English pronunciation. *Calorie* and *chronaxie*, though coined from Latin and Greek respectively, owe their spelling to French. *Frambesia* (in Europe, *framboesia*) is not Latin but a fabrication from French *framboise* = *raspberry*, which is in turn a corruption of a Germanic word, *brambusia*.

The expression *id reaction* has come into English by way of French also. Classical Greek employed the ending *–ides* as a patronymic: *Atrides (Atreides)* = *son of Atreus*. Latinized and pluralized, this suffix appears in the ending of family names: *Trypanosomidae, Culicidae*. In the nineteenth century it entered into the coinage of several French dermatologic terms, such as *syphilide* and *tuberculide*. Next it was taken into English, shorn of its final *e*, and added to a variety of stems with the generic meaning of *a skin condition due to* (e.g., *dermatophytid*). Finally, the suffix was given independent status as a word meaning an allergic dermatitis occurring at a site remote from that exposed to the allergen. (Freud's *id*, incidentally, is the Latin pronoun meaning *it*.) The living suffix *–ase*, regularly used to form the names of enzymes, first appeared in *diastase*, an eighteenth-century French coinage which is simply a Gallic rendering of Greek *diastasis* = *separation*.

From the Arabic alchemists we have inherited several words related to chemistry and pharmacy: *alcohol, elixir, sugar* and *syrup*. The Arabic *al qaliy* = *ashes* gives us both *alkali* and *kalium*, whence the symbol K for potassium. *Natron* is the source of *natrium* and the symbol *Na* for sodium. We are indebted to Arabic also for *arsenic, antimony* and perhaps *boron*. *Bezoar* (ultimately from Persian) was formerly a pharmacal term, too; it means *antidote*, and was applied to concretions found in the stomachs of animals, which were believed to have the power to neutralize poisons.

As an instance of how phonetic changes come about in borrowed words, the Arabic *luban jawi* = *frankincense of Java* was rendered *benzoi* by the Italians in the fifteenth century. They apparently dropped the first syllable from the noun because it sounded to them like their definite article *lo*, and since they had no *j* sound they substituted a *z*. By the middle of the seventeenth century, English, in common with most other European languages, had adopted the modern form *benzoin* for the natural substance. Around 1800 the chemical term *benzoic* was coined, whence later *benzine, benzol* and the numerous names of the *benzene* series.

Arabic *qahwah*, by way of Turkish *kahveh* and French *café*, has given us *caffeine*, the alkaloid of *coffee*. Interstingly, the Arabic word refers to the drink but not to the plant.

Names of diseases and drugs from distant countries often have an exotic lilt. Italian has contributed *belladonna, influenza, malaria, petechia* and *scarlatina*, while *cascara, espundia, marijuana, pinta* and *dengue* have come to us from Spanish, though the last was probably originally a Swahili word. Several other medical terms are derived ultimately from African languages: the *tsetse* fly is so called in Bechuana, and *kwashiorkor* means *displaced child* in the language of Ghana. The medicinal virtues of strophanthus were first noted in French Somaliland, and *ouabain* is a Gallicized spelling of *wabayo* (2), the native Somali name for the plant. *Ainhum* is a Portuguese version of the Yoruba (Nigerian) word *ayun=to saw or cut. Albino*, whence *albinism*, is also Portuguese.

Indic languages have contributed *kala-azar* (Assamese for *black disease*) and *beriberi* (Sinhalese *baeri=weakness;* the repetition adds emphasis: *great* weakness). The Hindustani word for a native washerman appears in *dhobie itch*.

From Japanese we have borrowed *tsutsugamushi=dangerous bug* and *sodoku*, which is adapted from Canton Chinese *shué=rat* and *tûk =poison.* Japanese *urushi=lacquer* is the source of the term *urushiol* for irritant substances from plants of the *Rhus* genus.

Curare, guanine, ipecac and *quinine* are derived from South American Indian words; so perhaps is *alastrim*, though it may be from Portuguese *alastrar=to scatter. Guaiacum* and its derivatives, from Spanish *guayaco*, are descended ultimately from a native Haitian word.

References to Literature and Mythology

*I beg leave to ask the candid reader, how he can prove to
me that all the heroes and heroines that have made him
hope, fear, admire, hate, love, shed tears, and laugh till
his sides were ready to burst, in novels and poems, are not
in possession of as perfect credentials of their existence as*

2. The French have neither a *w* in their alphabet nor an initial *w* sound in their language. The nearest they come to it is the sound of *ou* in *oui*, and accordingly this diphthong is often used to represent the initial *w* sound in words of non-French origin, as in *ouest* for Germanic *west*, *oued* for Arabic *wadi.*

the fattest of us? Common physical palpability is only a
proof of mortality.

James Leigh Hunt
***Men, Women, and Books** (3)*

Works of literature become classics because they are able to cap-
ture the imagination and engage the sympathies of readers of every
capacity and temperament by touching the most sensitive and most
universal chords of human nature. It is not surprising that some of the
heroes of world literature have become as familiar and real as historical
personages, and that we refer to them in our daily speech and writing.
Everyone who understands English is expected to know that a Jekyll-
Hyde personality is a changeable one, that a Scrooge is a miser, and that
a Frankenstein's monster is an experiment or enterprise gone awry (if
not amok).

The Spaniard sallies resolutely forth with Don Quixote or rattles
off hackneyed aphorisms with Sancho Panza; the German weeps with
Werther; and the Frenchman drinks deep from the cup of life with
Gargantua, Pantagruel and Panurge. Most genuine classics of western
literature have an international currency: witness the English adjectives
quixotic and *gargantuan,* the latter an antithesis to our home grown
lilliputian.

As in the general language, so in medicine we use names borrowed
from literature. A patient who repeatedly seeks medical attention for
nonexistent illnesses without any obvious ulterior motive is said to
display the *Munchausen "syndrome,"* a reference to the eighteenth century German cavalry officer Karl Friedrich Hieronymus, Baron von
Münchhausen. A collection of fantastic hunting and travel stories attributed to the Baron was published in England in 1785 by Rudolph
Erich Raspe, a wily rogue who had fled from the Continent to escape
imprisonment for fraud. The latter circumstance lends weight to the
theory that the real Baron never told any of the whoppers that Raspe
laid at his door.

The *Pickwick,* or *Pickwickian, syndrome* (pulmonary alveolar hypoventilation associated with corpulence) takes its name from Charles
Dickens' PICKWICK PAPERS, but does not refer to the corpulent Mr.
Pickwick himself. Pickwick's friend Mr. Wardle, a fine old country
gentleman, is invariably accompanied by a servant whose given name

3. Hunt L: MEN, WOMEN, AND BOOKS. NY, Harper & Brothers, 1860. Current
edition: NY, Gordon Press

is Joe but who is usually called simply "the fat boy." This indolent and somewhat mischievous lad has the remarkable ability to fall asleep as soon as he stops moving, even when he is on his feet. The only two things that seem able to rouse him are the smell of food and Mr. Wardle's good-natured observation, often repeated, *"Damn* the boy, he's fallen asleep again!"

Perhaps by analogy with this literary reference, pulmonary alveolar hypoventilation without corpulence has been called *Ondine's curse* or the *Ondine "syndrome"* after the water-nymph Undine of medieval German and Scandinavian folklore. The legend of Undine has furnished material for many fictional and dramatic works, including a 1939 play by Jean Giraudoux, whence the French spelling with initial *O*. According to one version of the legend (not, however, Giraudoux's, which is based on a nineteenth-century novella by Friedrich de la Motte-Fouqué) any mortal who fell in love with the nymph was doomed to a perpetual state of lethargy.

Every professional nurse knows that Sarah (or Sairy) Gamp is the embodiment of all that a nurse should not be, but few seem to be aware that the bibulous Mrs. Gamp never existed in fact. She is another of Charles Dickens' characters, and appears in MARTIN CHUZZLEWIT.

From a very different kind of literature, the Holy Bible, are derived the fanciful *Adam's apple* and the often misapplied *onanism.* Several popular hospital names are derived from Biblical narratives. On *Mount Sinai* God gave Moses the tables of the Law (Exodus, 19); Solomon built his temple with the wood of the *cedars of Lebanon* (I Kings, 5:6). The parable of the *good Samaritan* appears in Luke, 10:-30–37, and the health-restoring pool of *Bethesda* is described in John, 5:2–4.

It has been observed more than once that the *caput Medusae* is invariably found in textbooks of physical diagnosis, but very seldom in patients. The condition, not less spectacular than rare, takes its name from the Medusa of Roman mythology, whose head bore a tangle of snakes instead of hair.

Until the early part of the present century, a nodding acquaintance with the principal figures of Greek and Roman mythology was *de rigueur* for anyone with the least pretension to education and culture. Thus it is that such everyday words as *January, jovial, martial, Saturday, siren, tantalize* and *volcano* have come down to us from the preposterous superstitions of two civilizations that had collapsed a thousand years before the discovery of America.

Medical terminology contains many references to classic mythology. In anatomy, the otic *labyrinth* recalls the subterranean maze on the island of Crete, to the center of which Theseus penetrated to slay the Minotaur. Venus the love goddess is commemorated in *mons Veneris* as well as in *venereal disease.* The *tendo Achillis* refers to the one vulnerable spot of the Greek hero in the ILIAD. *Atlas,* who bore the world on his shoulders, has given his name to the first cervical vertebra.

The dermatitis seen around the necks of workers exposed to flying sparks is called the *collar of Vulcan* after the Olympian blacksmith. *Lethargy* is related to the *waters of Lethe,* which in Greek mythology induced forgetfulness. *Morphine* is named after the god of sleep, *atropine* after one of the three Fates, who was believed to cut off a person's thread of life at the moment appointed for him to die. *Fatal,* now synonymous with *deadly,* is another reference to the Fates.

Narcissism recalls the handsome youth who fell in love with his reflection in the water. From the lecherous tribe of Satyrs comes *satyriasis* and from Priapus, a fertility god, *priapism.* The myth of *Oedipus* is almost as widely known as the complex named after it. Proteus, who was able to change his appearance at will, has given us the adjective *protean,* referring to a disease of variable symptoms and signs, and also the bacterial genus name *Proteus.*

Arachne, Hygieia, Hymen, Iris and the Sphinx were mythical figures whose names were derived from the words that gave us *arachnidism, hygiene, hymen, iris* and *sphincter. Hermaphroditism* is named after the son of Hermes and Aphrodite, whose body became fused with that of a nymph so that it possessed physical features of both sexes. *Siren* and the *Cyclops* are also commemorated in teratology. The name of Hebe, goddess of youth, appears in *hebephrenic* and *ephebiatrics.*

Both the Aesculapian staff and the wand of Mercury often mistaken for it have their origins in mythology. The former, with one snake, is properly the symbol of medicine and healing. The latter, also known as the caduceus, has two snakes and also a pair of wings. Though it is the symbol of the medical corps in the various United States Armed Forces, it has no other connection with medicine.

Ammonia was first extracted from *sal ammoniac,* a salt collected near the Libyan city of Ammonia, which was named for the shrine of Jupiter Ammon built there. The *Rh factor* was first studied in a species of macaque named after Rhesus, a legendary king of Thrace.

Geographic Terms

I find that medicinal plants are named in various
ways . . . Some have retained the name of the region from

> *which they were formerly imported; so Median apples are
> called after Media, where they were first found; Punic
> apples, or pomegranates, are brought from Punicia,
> which we call Carthage; ligusticum, commonly known as
> lovage, is imported from Liguria in Italy; rhubarb gets its
> name from the River Rha in Barbary—at least that is
> Ammianus' contention; and we may add santonica, fenu-
> greek, persicaria and a whole host of others.*
>
> François Rabelais
> ***Gargantua and Pantagruel, Book Third***

The application of place-names to common things is a practice of great antiquity. In the ancient world the finest paper obtainable was that made at Pergamon in Asia Minor (the birthplace of Galen), and so this paper came to be known simply as *pergamon,* of which our word *parchment* is a corruption. *Bayonet, coach, copper, gauze, peach* and *wiener* are among the many other words in English that are derived from place-names.

In medical terminology, too, we find many geographic allusions. Though most of them are straightforward, like *Aleppo boil* or *Zanzibar swelling,* in some instances the original form of the place-name is lost. For example, *vernix,* a medieval Latin word used unchanged in obstetric parlance and in the corrupted form *varnish* in the vernacular, was derived, by way of an intermediate term *veronice,* from *Berenike,* a city of Cyrenaicum where the first varnish was prepared. Before its nature was elucidated, the disease caused by *Coxiella burnetii* was named Q (for *query*) *fever;* afterwards the name stuck because it had acquired an association with the state of Queensland, Australia.

In the nineteenth chapter of Genesis is recounted the destruction of the iniquitous Cities of the Plain by fire and brimstone; one of them, Sodom, has given its name to *sodomy.* The *risus sardonicus* of tetany and strychnine poisoning (whence our common English adjective *sardonic*) is a reference to Sardinia, because it was first noted as an effect of poisoning by a plant that grew in that island. Though this may have been the nux vomica from which strychnine has been produced in modern times, it was probably another plant of the *Strychnos* genus, or perhaps even an altogether different herb.

Epsom salts are named after an English town in the county of Surrey, whose long-famous mineral waters owe their medicinal effect chiefly to a high concentration of magnesium sulfate. *Magnesium,* incidentally, is named after the city of Magnesia in Thessaly. The five-carbon sugar *arabinose* gets its name from Arabia, by way of *gum arabic,* while *indole* is derived, both chemically and etymologically, from *indigo,* a dyestuff from India.

Because the epicanthal folds of children with certain genetic abnormalities gave their faces an Asiatic configuration (in the view of western observers) they were dubbed *mongoloid.* The lay term for conjoined twins is *Siamese,* after Chang and Eng, who were born in Siam in 1811 and were for many years a major attraction in P. T. Barnum's sideshows.

Thalassemia, from classical Greek *thalassa = the sea,* is another name for Mediterranean anemia, a congenital hemolytic disorder affecting particularly the races inhabiting the Mediterranean littoral.

We have noted that syphilis was known in the sixteenth century as *morbus Gallicus = the French disease.* This expression seems to have been in general use in most European countries except France, where the affliction was commonly fathered on the Spanish. Occasionally even in English writings of the time there is reference to the *Spanish pox.* Nor were the French the only ones to refer to the influenza pandemic of 1918 as *Spanish influenza;* that expression was usual in the United States, though the British preferred *Flanders grippe.* A list of the important influenza outbreaks of the past half-century reads like the itinerary of an incurable wanderer. Even more cosmopolitan are the many *Salmonella* species.

Quite a few American place-names have found their way into the terminology of medicine. *Haverhill fever* is named after the city in Massachusetts, and nearby Boston gives its name to *Boston exanthem.* Coccidioidomycosis is also known as *San Joaquin Valley fever* after the region of the Southwest where it is endemic. *Rocky Mountain spotted fever* is unfortunately not so limited in distribution as the name suggests. *Tularemia* and *Pasteurella tularensis* are named after Tulare County, California. American geographic names are found also in the *Milwaukee brace* for scoliosis, *Chicago disease* (a synonym for North American blastomycosis) and *St. Louis encephalitis.*

Eponyms

Some medicinal herbs bear the name of him who first discovered them, cultivated them, or investigated and published their virtues; thus mercuriale, from Mercury; panacea, from Panace, the daughter of Aesculapius; armois, from Artemis, also called Diana; eupatoria, from

> *King Eupator; euphorbium, from Euphorbius, physician*
> *to King Juba; clymenos, from Clymenus; alcibiadon, from*
> *Alcibiades; and gentian, from Gentius, King of Scla-*
> *vonia.*
>
> François Rabelais
> **Gargantua and Pantagruel, Book Third**

Just as occupational designations like *baker* and *cartwright* have often been borrowed from the English language and applied to particular persons as proper names, so the names of particular persons sometimes become common nouns. *Blanket, boycott, derrick, dunce, leotard, sandwich, shrapnel,* and *silhouette* are all men's names.

In medicine we do not often go so far as to spell eponyms with a small letter, though there are a few exceptions, like *condom* and *scultetus bandage.* We do, however, form out of proper names a great many compound words spelled with small initial letters: *bartholinectomy, chagoma, descemetocele, galenical, graafian, marfanoid, pagetic, parkinsonism, politzerize, roentgenogram, skenitis, voltage.*

Species designations in Linnaean taxonomy are spelled with small initial letters even when derived from proper names. Most of these eponymous species designations have been Latinized and put into the genitive (possessive) case. Because the endings *–us* and *–ius* are used indiscriminately in Latinizing proper names, the genitives may terminate in either one or two *i*'s. Examples of this variability are seen in the species names of the *Rickettsiae: mooseri* and *parkeri* as contrasted with *ricketsii* and *prowazekii.*

Genus names are of course spelled with a capital letter whether eponymous or not. The endings *–ia* (less often *–a*) and *–ella* (less often *–iella*) are used to convert proper names into genus names: *Rauwolfia, Leishmania, Gaffkya, Brucella, Pasteurella, Klebsiella. Nicotiana* (whence *nicotine*) and *Sabouraudites* are pleasant variations from the usual pattern.

Eponyms have been called tombstone words. In recent years there has been a strong tendency to expunge proper names from the working vocabulary of the medical profession. There are, however, a few exceptions to this general trend: *Hansen's disease* and *Down's syndrome* have been promoted as euphemisms for, respectively, leprosy and mongolism.

Certainly the student of anatomy associates *uterine tube* more readily than *fallopian tube* with the uterus. In medicine we have no such fortuitously appropriate eponyms as the Pullman railroad car or the

Bell telephone (though the term *bel* and its more familiar derivative *decibel* do commemorate Alexander Graham Bell). But even apart from the lack of any logical relationship between an eponym and the thing named, proper names themselves generate a great deal of confusion.

What American physician has not puzzled over the correct pronunciation of *Chvostek, Kveim* and *Sjögren?* *Lutembacher* and *Gaucher,* though often given German pronunciations, are French names, whereas *eustachian,* generally pronounced with a soft French *ch,* refers to an Italian anatomist, and *Behçet* is not French but Turkish. (Gallicization of medical terms is a fad that refuses to die, and has spread far beyond the eponyms. We shall see more of it in Chapter 7.) The developer of *Burow's* solution was German, though Americans seem irresistibly tempted to make him an English Burrows or Burroughs.

Absurdities like *collagen's disease, caisson's disease,* and *planter's wart* are unfortunately not confined to the laity, though *Emerson's* (for *emesis*) *basin, charcoal* (for *Charcot*) *joints,* and *change-strokes* (for *Cheyne-Stokes*) *breathing* probably are.

Other languages than English have their share of these phonetic errors. To a German, *Kussmaul respiration* sounds positively ludicrous, for *Kussmaul* means *kiss-mouth.* The renowned German clinician who bore this name used to introduce himself to each new class of medical students with the remark that there were more than seventy possible puns on *Kussmaul,* and that any student who wanted to save himself the trouble of thinking them up could buy a printed set from one of the upperclassmen.

The *coudé* catheter was not designed by Dr. Coudé: the word is French for *bent.* On the other hand, the *Sippy diet* was devised by Dr. Bertram Sippy, and the *Quick Prothrombin Time Test,* though it can indeed be done more quickly than the two-stage test, was named after its originator, Dr. Armand Quick. The *corpora Arantii* of the cardiac valves are not *orange bodies* (as if dog-Latin *aurantia,* the issue of an irregular union between Latin *aurum=gold* and Arabic *naranj=an orange*) but the *bodies of Arantius* (Italian anatomist Giulio Aranzi).

A compound eponym may refer to more than one person *(Hand-Schüller-Christian, Laurence-Moon-Biedl)* or may be a double name borne by a single person, as in the case of *Brown-Sequard* and *Parkes-Weber* (with a hyphen) and *Ramsay Hunt* and *Graham Steell* (without).

In a few instances, the same name is attached to two or more diseases, and we are then obliged to distinguish: Paget's disease of the nipple, Paget's disease of bone; von Recklinghausen's disease of bone, von Recklinghausen's disease of skin.

Despite frequent misplacement of the apostrophe, Chagas,

Coombs, Graves, Homans and Meigs all spelled their names with a final *s*. The use of the *'s* has never been consistent, and the modern trend is to do away with it altogether.

As in the case of *derrick* and *sandwich,* we often drop out the qualified noun and use the proper name to stand for the thing itself. A *Kelly hemostat* is usually just a *Kelly,* and few physicians take the time to say or write *Foley catheter* or *Babinski sign.* In "Diarrhea due to Sonne is seldom as severe as that caused by Flexner," the speaker is comparing *Shigella sonnei* dysentery with that caused by *S. flexneri.*

Some eponyms are customarily abbreviated beyond recognition. Only the first syllable of the name of George Papanicolaou, the pioneer in cervical cytology, is preserved in *Pap smear,* which, moreover, is often written with a small *p.* The names of the German microbiologist Escherich and the American pathologist Salmon are usually whittled down to single letters in common usage: *E.* (for *Escherichia*) *coli* and *S.* (for *Salmonella*) *paratyphi.* Hartnup disease is often simply *H disease.* Other abbreviations that conceal eponyms are *NPH insulin (neutral protamine, Hagedorn)* and *BCG vaccine (bacillus of Calmette and Guérin.)*

A medical eponym does not necessarily refer to the physician or scientist who discovered or first described the thing named. This is especially noticeable in the case of taxonomic terms, which are often chosen to honor famous public figures. *Serratia* is named after Serafino Serrati, who (according to the Italians) invented the steamship. *Listeria* is named in honor of Lord Lister, the nineteenth-century developer of aseptic surgery, who was long dead before the genus named after him was discovered. The brand name *Listerine,* however, was coined in his lifetime, and he spent a great deal of money, unsuccessfully, to suppress the term, which seemed to link him with a proprietary product that had no connection with him or his work.

Sadism and *masochism* are named after two novelists, the French Count (usually called Marquis) de Sade and the Austrian Leopold von Sacher-Masoch, in whose works these perversions were described. *Christmas disease* was first identified in a patient whose surname was Christmas. The *Musset sign,* a rhythmic nodding of the head seen in aortic regurgitation, is named for the French poet and novelist Alfred de Musset, who was so afflicted. *Daltonism,* a now archaic name for color-blindness, refers to the English physicist John Dalton, the originator of the modern atomic theory, whose inability to distinguish colors occasionally led to his wearing clothing whose hues scandalized his fellow Quakers. *Pott's fracture* is named after the English surgeon Percivall Pott, who developed a method of treating bimalleolar ankle fracture after himself suffering such an injury. *Carrión's disease* takes its name from the young South American bacteriologist who elucidated the nature of the disease by inoculating himself with it—an experiment that proved fatal. *Rickettsia prowazekii,* the organism that causes epidemic typhus, claimed the lives of both Ricketts and von Prowazek.

Among older eponyms we encounter some very distinguished names. The *caesarean section* has traditionally been traced to Julius Caesar, who was allegedly delivered in this way. *Chorea* was formerly *chorea Sancti Viti=St. Vitus' dance,* after the martyr whose intercession was believed able to cure the affliction, and erysipelas was once called *St. Anthony's fire* for a similar reason. *Stensen's duct* is named after a seventeenth century Danish anatomist who was also a Roman Catholic bishop. *Cretinism* seems to have been derived from the name of Christ, though the exact etymology is obscure.

5

modern coinages, abbreviations, and trade names

Modern Coinages

When things newly discovered demand terms newly framed to express them clearly, there is no objection to the coinage of words, provided that the process is carried out with judgment and taste . . . Words of recent fabrication always find ready acceptance when they are built out of Greek material.

Horace
The Art of Poetry

The position of Latin as the *lingua franca* of western scholars in the post-Renaissance world was a major reason why the nomenclature of the developing physical sciences was fundamentally Latin and Latinized Greek. But there was a second and no less cogent reason: though Latin was a universal medium of communication among the learned, it was a "dead" language; not only was it nobody's mother tongue, but it was little more amenable to alteration or corruption through use than, say, the Morse code.

Latin afforded a vast fund of words to which specific technical meanings could be assigned arbitrarily without generating confusion with other usages. The early anatomists found it more practical to build up a nomenclature consisting of words like *femur, ilium, acetabulum* and *gluteus* than to assign any one of these meanings arbitrarily and exclusively to the word *hip,* which in vernacular use could mean any of them, or all of them collectively. Moreover, Latin and Greek were gold-mines of root words and affixes from which the scientist could fashion new terms that, if not altogether self-explanatory, could at least be readily understood and remembered by any educated person.

These principles apply today just as truly as they did four centuries ago, and whether we like it or not we are obliged to retain a cumbersome and foreign-seeming terminology consisting of borrowings and coinages from dead languages—deader than ever now that they no longer form an integral part of secondary education. Some notion of the difficulty of changing to a new terminology may be gained by a consideration of the extreme slowness with which authoritative revisions in nomenclature are learned, accepted, and adopted by the medical profession. The *eustachian tube* and the *fallopian tube* were both officially laid to rest a generation ago, yet they still flourish in daily speech, and even in journal articles and textbooks. The genus names *Staphylococcus* and *Streptococcus* live on despite the attempts of Bergey and others to substitute *Micrococcus* as long ago as 1948.

Nevertheless, a strong case can be made against the continued coinage of new terms from Latin and Greek. Many younger physicians have not acquired even a smattering of either in the course of their studies, and most older ones have long ago forgotten their classic languages along with their trigonometry and ancient history. Indeed, coiners of new words themselves often go astray in their choice of material. *Sphygmos,* as in *sphygmomanometer,* means not *pressure* but *pulse* (from *sphygein = to throb*). Though Laënnec's original stethoscope was a jointed wooden tube, he was scarcely justified in making it a brother to the telescope, for it was used to listen to, not look at, the chest *(stethos = chest; scopein = to look at).* In a journal article on the hyperlipidemias we find reference to the *infranatant* plasma. This adjective was no doubt fabricated by analogy with the well-established *supernatant* (from Latin *super = above* and *natans = swimming*). But if the lipid layer is *supernatant* (swimming above) and the plasma is *infranatant* (swimming below), the question arises just what it is that the two are swimming in.

There would seem to be no objection to the continued use of stems whose meaning is familiar because they already appear in other words of wide use. Thus, no physician will have any difficulty in deciphering *atherogenicity* or *hypomagnesemia* the first time he encounters them. On the other hand, who recognizes that *fulguration* comes from Latin *fulgur = lightning,* or that *botulism* is derived from *botulus = sausage?*

Even some well-known stems are limited in usefulness by the inconsistency with which they are applied. The family of *–philias,* for example, is a variegated collection of terms formed upon several different models. In *necrophilia* we see the Greek word in its literal meaning, *love or attraction. Hemophilia,* however, cannot be considered an analogous use except by the exercise of considerable imagination. *Argyrophilia* and *basophilia* are metaphorical extensions of the notion of attraction; but *eosinophilia* and *neutrophilia* are in present-day use far more often applied not to the cells whose cytoplasmic granules show affinity for eosin and neutral stains, but to conditions in which the numbers of these cells in the blood are increased.

Medical dictionaries contain whole dynasties of *-emias, -penias, -oses, -urias* and *-algias,* in each of which the stem word has several loosely related meanings. As we have already observed elsewhere, half a dozen different significations may be tortured out of a single stem like *gen-* or *path-.* Among twentieth-century inventions we have the large and motley family of *-pathies. Adenopathy* means "something wrong with the glands"; *neuropathy,* "something wrong with a nerve"; *uropathy,* "something wrong with the excretory system." Each of these terms labors under the double disadvantage of vagueness in meaning coupled with an illusory flavor of specificity.

But for that very reason they are handy words for the intellectually indolent, and the *-pathy* clan shows no signs of dying out. Indeed, we now have *vasculopathy, cardiomyopathy,* and even *coagulopathy.* Ironically, *empathy* has become a fad word for *sympathy,* though it was coined expressly to signify something different from sympathy. *Empathy* is a "translation" of German *Einfühlung,* which means intellectual insight into another's emotional state without any sharing of feelings. A distant cousin of the *-pathy* family is the adjective *idiopathic.* The original Greek word, formed from *idios=personal, private* and *pathos=disease,* was applied by Galen to any disease that arises of itself in the part affected. Though modern scientific medicine tells us that there is no such thing, the word continues to be used for conditions whose origin modern scientific medicine has yet to explain. In this context some physicians seem to take the term *idiopathic* as a personal affront, as though it connoted a disease that the doctor is "too much of an idiot to explain," and have opted for the equally unscientific and noncommittal adjective *essential: essential hypertension, essential hypoglycemia.*

A great many classical stems used in scientific terminology have completely lost their original meanings and acquired new ones by association or analogy. *Autopsy* means a personal inspection—seeing for oneself, from *autos=self* and *opsis=view.* But as the word came to refer specifically to a dissection and pathologic examination of a dead body, it seemed proper to form a new term for removal of living tissue for pathologic examination by introducing the stem *bi-,* from *bios=life: biopsy.*

Classic Greek used several suffixes to turn verbs into nouns, as we do with *-ation, -ance* and *-ment*. One of these was *-ismos*, by the addition of which *ptyalizein=to salivate* becomes *ptyalismos=the act of salivating*. Many medical terms both ancient and modern owe their origins to this process, including *bruxism* (derived, a little irregularly, from classical *brychismos*), *metabolism* and *organism*.

The suffix *-ismos*, generally Anglicized to *-ism* but occasionally appearing in the Latinized form *-ismus*, is a living affix in the general language, where it is used to name doctrines *(Buddhism)*, theories *(behaviorism)*, personal traits *(altruism)*, states of mind *(pessimism)* and statements or expressions *(Maoism, truism)*. Curiously, most of its roles in the language of medicine bear no relation to these patterns. In medicine, *-ism* can be used to form eponymous disease names *(parkinsonism)*, to denote intoxications *(atropinism, ethanolism, loxoscelism)*, and indeed to indicate any abnormal state *(meningism, prostatism)*. Perhaps by mistaken identification with *tenesmus=painful straining to void or defecate* and *trismus* (Greek *trigmos*)*=painful spasm of the jaw muscles*, the meaning of *laryngismus* shifted from the literal sense, *the act of shouting*, to *spasm of the vocal cords*. It was evidently on this same model that Sims, in the 1860s, fashioned the term *vaginismus*.

The suffix *-asis* was another means of turning a Greek verb into a noun: *histasthai=to stand* yields *stasis=a standing*. It is interesting to review the stages through which *-asis* has passed to reach its modern role as a living suffix for naming infestations. To form *phthiriasis= infestation with lice* from the noun *phthir=louse*, the Greeks had first to coin a verb, *phthirian=to be infested with lice*. Similarly, *lithiasis* implies an intermediate verb meaning *to become stony*, and *elephantiasis*, a very old word, implies a verb meaning *to become like an elephant*. Perhaps through the example of the latter word, the modern term *filariasis* was invented to mean *infestation with filariae*. Note that the stem word here ends in *-ia*, and that the entire word *filaria* is preserved within the derived form. Next we find other *i*-stem words like *Balantidium* forming derivatives like *balantidiasis*, in which only the *i* of the stem is preserved. Finally, words with no *i* at the end of their stems, such as *Candida, Paragonimus*, and *Trichomonas*, form derivatives in which the *i* is nonetheless supplied so that all members of the family will match up in sound: *candidiasis, paragonimiasis, trichomoniasis*.

Yet another termination employed by the Greeks to form a noun from a verb was *-oma*, as in *scotoma*, from *scotoun=to darken*. Its appearance in *sarcoma* (from *sarcoun=to become fleshy)* and *condyloma* (from *condylomai=to become knobby*) has led to its adoption as a generic ending for the name of any kind of tumor or abnormal mass whatever, and we now have a long list of derivatives, in which the stem word may indicate the site of the tumor *(hepatoma, hypernephroma)*, its histologic type *(epithelioma)*, its biochemical composition *(atheroma, cholesteatoma)*, the substance it produces *(insulinoma, glucagonoma)*, the causative microorganism *(ameboma)* or even the eponym attached to the tissue of origin *(schwannoma)*.

The suffix *–gram* has achieved great popularity as an all-purpose ending for the name of a diagnostic procedure. Originally from Greek *graphein = to write, –gram* appeared first in *electrocardiogram* and *electroencephalogram,* in which a sort of writing is in fact present. Next the termination was applied to a variety of x-ray examinations *(renogram, arteriogram, tomogram),* and finally its meaning was extended even to laboratory study of the blood cells *(hemogram).*

Besides making extensive use of suffixes like these, modern medical terminology freely forms new words by addition of prefixes, most of them prepositions borrowed more or less intact from the classical languages. The Greek *a–(alpha privative) = without* appears in literally hundreds of technical words. When the word or stem to which it is prefixed begins with a vowel, it resumes its original form, *an–,* as in *anisocytosis* and *anencephalic.* This *an–* is not to be confused with *ana–,* an unrelated preposition meaning *up to,* as in *anabolic* and *anasarca.* In *atrophy* and *apnea* the prefixed *a* is usually pronounced as in *cat;* in *aphasia* and *anemia,* as in *canoe;* and in *achlorhydria* and *asystole,* as in *cake.*

The Greek preposition *anti = against* is seldom confused with Latin *ante = before,* though they are generally given identical pronunciations. Similarly, Greek *peri = around* and Latin *per = through* maintain a peaceful coexistence without the least friction or confusion. *Peri* is occasionally confounded with *para,* because in words like *perineum* and *peritoneum* the *i* tends to be slurred into a neutral vowel sound much like the second *a* in *para.*

Pro in Latin is nearly identical in meaning with Greek *pro,* but the Latin preposition most closely analogous to Greek *pro* is *prae,* which in English compounds is usually shortened to *pre–.* This word originally meant *in front of* but eventually took on the additional meaning *earlier than.* For some reason it is especially liable to abuse. If pretibial edema is in front of the shinbones, then *presacral* edema should be in front of the sacrum, which would make its detection very difficult indeed. And surely it is pointless to refer to disseminated intravascular coagulation as a *preterminal* event when in fact every event in life comes *before the end. Pre-mortem* is not only a superfluous affectation but it is wrong thrice over: 1) The use of an oblique case makes it clear that this is a Latin phrase, not an English coinage, and therefore the preposition should be spelled *prae.* 2) In a prepositional phrase the hyphen is out of place. 3) Since *prae* takes the ablative case, *mortem* (no doubt borrowed from *post mortem*) should be *morte*. But the correct literary antithesis of *post mortem* is *ante mortem*.

A few of the prefixes that are not prepositions are particularly susceptible to being stretched out of all conformity to common sense. Latin *semis* means *half,* and retains that meaning in older compounds like *semilunar* and *semitendinosus*. Since the fourteenth century, though, it has been customary to apply this prefix in the extremely broad sense of *somewhat, partly, incompletely* or *almost,* and we now have *semicomatose, semisynthetic, semi-Fowler's position* and even *semi-intensive care unit!*

Quasi=as if also appears in a number of loose and inconsistent applications, such as *quasi-diagnostic procedure, quasi-murmur,* and *quasi-splint*. We even read, in a book review, that the author has made a "quasi-Flexner request for improving the quality of American surgery." Another affix of variable purport is *dys-,* which in modern medical terminology may mean painful *(dyspareunia),* difficult *(dyspnea),* abnormal *(dysgenesis),* or *lack of (dyssynergia).* In *dysuria* its meaning vacillates, in common usage, between *difficult* and *painful.*

The medical profession has great fun with the prefix *pseudo-,* from the Greek verb meaning *to deceive.* A *pseudo-Cushing's syndrome,* one would suppose, is a syndrome described by a bogus Dr. Harvey Cushing. As if *pseudohypoparathyroidism* were not sufficiently lengthy and intricate, a similar condition has actually been named *pseudo-pseudohypoparathyroidism. Pseudalgia,* literally *false pain,* positively defies semantic analysis.

Not all modern coinages are compounds formed of two or more stems, or of stems and affixes. Examples of terms formed from single stems include *moron, sol, gel, ion, proton, neutron* and *electron.* But as most fabricated words involve some kind of marriage between words or word fragments, a few remarks on this process are in order.

The combination of a Greek with a Latin stem in the same word was formerly regarded as a serious breach of linguistic decorum, and such hybrids were called bastard words. According to this view, *chloroform, hypertension, monocular, neutrophil, radiology* and *retinitis* are vulgar amalgamations, to be eschewed by cultivated speakers and writers.

In the days when every educated person knew a good deal of Latin and at least a little Greek, physicians made a sincere effort to avoid improper conjunctions of the two, and that is no doubt the reason why we have so many duplications of stems in our present system of terminology. *Subungual* is pure Latin *(sub=under* and *unguis=nail).* To coin a word meaning *loosening of the nail* by combining *unguis* with

Greek *lysis* would formerly have been unthinkable, and so the Greek word for *nail, onyx,* was pressed into service: *onycholysis.*

But surely a prejudice against intermixing various language stocks in the formation of new words is slightly ridiculous in speakers of English, which is of all languages ever spoken the most various in origin. Fortunately, this species of pedantic purism died out when classical studies began to disappear from the high school curriculum, and we can now talk of *periungual* warts without a qualm. As might be expected, the various Romance language academies, intent upon keeping their respective wells of Latin undefiled, continue to frown upon Greco–Latin hybrids. In Spanish, for example, even words of such international currency as *cablegrama* and *panamericano* are condemned as "defective," and their use discouraged.

A heated debate was carried on among physicians not many years ago over the term *progestogen,* which was a modification of *progesterone* intended to take its place alongside *estrogen* and *androgen.* The objection to this word was not that it contained both Latin and Greek elements (which it does) but that the second *o* had been wrongly substituted for the *a* in the stem of the Latin verb *gestare=to bear.* Though this may seem a formidable argument in favor of the alternate spelling *progestagen,* it is actually without any validity whatever.

The use of *o* to make combining forms of Latin and Greek stems is a practice dating back to remote antiquity. In classic Greek the *o* was employed regularly in the formation of compound words, regardless of stem vowels. The primitive pattern of such words is seen in *Acropolis,* where a noun, *polis=city,* is qualified by a combining form derived from an adjective *(akron=highest).* Very early the process was extended to nouns and verbs: *cardio–, osteo–, crypto–, schizo–.* Next the connecting *o* appeared in Latin, nearly replacing the older Latin connective, *i* (which is still seen, however, in a few words such as *unilateral* and *sensorimotor*).

The connecting *o* is a phonetic device of the kind favored by Mediterranean languages. With rare exceptions like *speedometer,* English does not use it in building compounds out of Anglo-Saxon stock, preferring to deal with native material in a more traditionally Germanic fashion. Even in Latin and Greek words the connective is omitted after prefixes *(en–, per–, dys–, pan–)* and applied only to noun and verb stems.

When the second element in a compound begins with a vowel, no connective ending need be attached to the first one: *arthr | algia, hemat | uria.* Hence not every *o* in the middle of a word is an inserted connective; in *pleurodynia,* for example, the *o* is provided by *odyne= pain,* and in *leuconychia* by *onyx=nail.*

The practice of discarding the stem vowel of a noun or verb and making a combining form end in *o* is not quite universal. The retention of the stem vowel by such irregular combining forms as *chole–, pyle–, genu–* and *manu–* rests on the authority of classic models. But as medical dictionaries contain thousands of words in which the connective *o* has been attached to *a*-stem nouns and verbs, it is hard to understand why *progestogen* aroused such a storm of protest. Though it may continue to grate like a rusty hinge on the ears of amateur classicists, it has won an easy victory over the spelling with *a*, which has long ago gone wherever bad words go when they die.

An oddity that has proven more durable is *neurilemma*. In the original word, *neurilema*, the *i* was contributed by the second member of the compound, *eilema = covering*. No sooner had the word been coined (in the early nineteenth century) than the variant spelling with two *m*'s was adopted by medical writers who mistakenly supposed the last two syllables to represent Greek *lemma = hull*. Were this the case, the word should properly be spelled *neurolemma*, but apparently these innovators were either not well enough informed or not sufficiently meddlesome to make the second change. The *e* of *venesection* is not an illegitimate connective but merely a corruption of the diphthong *ae* in the Latin phrase *venae sectio = cutting of a vein*, of which the English word is a composite.

Though the connective *o* can legitimately be substituted for any stem vowel, the final consonant of a stem is and should be carefully preserved. Many Latin and Greek nouns have different final consonants in oblique cases than they have in the nominative case: *pes, ped–; dens, dent–; hepar, hepat–; glottis, glottid–*. Latin words may undergo a vowel shift, with or without a change of final consonant: *glomus, glomer–; femur, femor–*. In building compounds with these words, or adding suffixes to them, we should be careful to use the genitive ("begetting") form, if it differs from the nominative. Though *iritis, myositis* and *sinusitis* are well-established variants, and are perhaps more euphonious than the "correct" forms, *iriditis, myitis* and *sinuitis*, there is no excuse for the continuing coinage of such barbarous monstrosities as *arachnitis, circadian, euthanize* and *serumcidality*.

There are, however, some instances in which a shortened version of a combining form may be perfectly serviceable. Derivatives of Greek *derma = skin* should properly be formed with *dermat–*, but the usual combining form (as in modern terms like *dermabrasion* and *dermographism*) omits the last syllable of the stem. Though THE OXFORD ENGLISH DICTIONARY coldly observes that such words are not formed on Greek analogies, and suggests that *dermatic* would be preferable to *dermal*, we find *dermopteros = leather-winged* in so ancient a work as Aristotle's HISTORY OF ANIMALS. *Hemo–*, *chromo–* and *teno–* are widely accepted shortenings of *hemato–*, *chromato–* and *tenonto–*. *Pneumo–* does double duty as the abbreviated version of two combining forms: *pneumato–*, referring to *air* or *breath (pneuma)*, and *pneumono–*, referring to the *lung (pneumon)*; compare *pneumothorax* and *pneumoconiosis*.

Plasmato– is usually shortened not to *plasmo–* but to the still more irregular *plasma–*, as in *plasmacyte, plasmapheresis*. But perhaps it would be both simpler and more accurate to regard *plasma–* as a combining form which, like *chole–* and *genu–*, preserves the final vowel of the nominative case instead of adding the connective *o* to the stem.

What is the difference between *boric* and *boracic?* Is the correct spelling *lymphangitis* or *lymphangiitis?* Careful speakers and writers are apt to look askance at the shorter form in each case, and to suspect that the dropping of a syllable is, if not absolutely erroneous, at least an innovation that smacks of carelessness.

Boracic is formed from *borax*, while the more modern *boric* comes from *boron*. The shorter form is now considered preferable, not only because it *is* shorter but also because it seems better to form a chemical name directly from the name of an element than from that of a crude substance. (In the elaboration of *formic* from *formica = ant* there was a short-lived intermediate term, *formicic*.)

The case of *dilatation–dilation* is altogether different. The second syllable of the verb *dilate* represents the Latin adjective *latus = wide;* it is not a passive participle ending like the *–late* of *ablate* and *correlate*. Unlike these latter, then, *dilate* cannot be turned into a noun by the conversion of *–late* into *–lation;* indeed, there is no such word as *dilation*, and the only proper noun form is *dilatation*.

Concerning technical words coined from Greek *angeion = vessel* there is no fixed rule for the extra syllable. Buerger's disease is almost invariably called *thromboangiitis obliterans*, whereas *cholangitis* is consistently spelled with a single *i*. The first *i* in *thromboangiitis* represents the diphthong *ei* in the Greek stem, and the second *i* is of course contributed by *–itis*. Whereas the *i* of the stem fits nicely into such words as *angioma* and *angiogram*, in which it is needed to preserve the soft sound of the *g* after *n*, it is neither necessary nor euphonious in *angiitis*. Though there are exceptions *(myofasciitis)*, the current trend seems to be to avoid repeating the *i* sound.

Choroid is an old corruption of *chorioid = resembling the chorion* (fetal membrane), but the *i* is preserved in the combining form *chorio–*. *Histology*, however, does not contain a defective form of the stem seen in *histiocyte*. The former word is built from *histos = web, tissue* and the latter from its diminutive *histion*. In many instances, of course, the inclusion of an additional syllable completely changes the meaning of a word. *Posthepatic* jaundice is a synonym for obstructive jaundice, but *posthepatitic* cirrhosis occurs *after hepatitis. Arteriosclerosis* is a generic term for a group of related vascular diseases, of which *arteriolosclerosis* is one.

In some terms of fairly recent coinage, an awkward syllable has been deliberately left out: *contraception* and *urinalysis* are much easier to say than *contraconception* and *urinanalysis*. By the process of haplology two identical-sounding syllables have been fused in *albumin* (*albumen* =*eggwhite* and –*in*, chemical suffix) and *cephalgia* (*cephale*=*head* and *algos*=*pain*). *Thoracentesis* and *appendectomy* are abbreviated forms of the older and more correct *thoracocentesis* and *appendicectomy;* the longer forms are still sometimes used in England.

𝔄𝔟𝔟𝔯𝔢𝔳𝔦𝔞𝔱𝔦𝔬𝔫𝔰

> *It is one thing to abbreviate by contracting, another by cutting off.*
>
> Francis Bacon
> *Essays, "Of Dispatch"*

In their sometimes desperate and usually fruitless efforts to conserve time, physicians have recourse to many abbreviations in speech and writing, which most often consist of the initials of the words in a phrase. *CBC*=*complete blood count, IV*=*intravenous(ly)* and *ENT*=*ear, nose and throat* not only are universally understood within the medical profession but are almost invariably substituted, even in print, for the full expressions.

Abbreviations are especially popular for the names of diseases and of diagnostic and therapeutic procedures: *ASHD*=*arteriosclerotic heart disease, SBE*=*subacute bacterial endocarditis, BUN*=*blood urea nitrogen, SGOT*=*serum glutamic-oxalacetic transaminase, IPPB*=*intermittent positive-pressure breathing,* and *BSO*=*bilateral salpingo-oophorectomy* are intelligible to every physician.

Though any of these might be printed in a journal article, there is another class of abbreviations that is seldom seen except in handwritten clinical records. *WDWNWM C/O SOB* would be readily translated by most American physicians as *well-developed and well-nourished white male complaining of shortness of breath. UCD*=*usual childhood diseases,*

PERLA = pupils are equal, react to light and accommodate, and *RCM = right costal margin* are nearly universal forms of shorthand.

Whereas these expressions are entirely unintelligible to the non-professional some abbreviations, like *BM = bowel movement* and *DOA = dead on arrival,* have found their way into the vernacular. A few such serve as euphemisms: *CA* for *cancer, VD* for *venereal disease.*

Some abbreviations arise from the need to compress a notation into a small space on a printed form, as when a laboratory technician performing a urinalysis writes, in the space provided for the number of white blood cells seen in a high-power field, *TNTC = too numerous to count,* or enters for the specific gravity *QNS = quantity not sufficient* (to float a hydrometer).

Though abbreviations are extremely serviceable, they have two disadvantages worth noting: they mean nothing whatever until they have been explained, and they may occasionally be dangerously ambiguous. A few years ago, if a drug-abuser admitted swallowing *THC,* the physician could reasonably conclude that he meant *terpin hydrate* (elixir) with *codeine;* nowadays the abbreviation *THC* is more likely to stand for $\Delta,9$-*tetrahydrocannabinol*(1). When a physician's admitting note indicates that the "Patient had PE 6 months ago," the fact may be reassuring or ominous depending on whether the *PE* was a *physical examination* or a *pulmonary embolism.*

Fortunately, the intended meaning is usually apparent from the context, and it seems unlikely that the three common meanings of *MS* (*morphine sulfate, multiple sclerosis, mitral stenosis*) or the three meanings of *BS* (*blood sugar, breath sounds, bowel sounds*) could often be confounded in practice. Nevertheless, most hospitals have found it advisable to standardize the abbreviations that physicians are permitted to use in writing orders.

A great many abbreviations in common use have lost all connection with their origins. *Streptolysin O* is so distinguished because it is inactivated by *oxygen,* but to a physician interested in his patient's antistreptolysin O titre, that fact is of no particular concern or use. *TB* was originally an abbreviation for *tubercle bacillus* but was quickly picked up by the laity as a euphemism for *tuberculosis.* In a similar way *GC* in modern professional parlance has come to stand not for *gonococcus* but for the disease it causes.

1. Not all of the confusion arising from abbreviations is purely linguistic. Pfeifer, in a letter to Drug Therapy (May, 1975, p 14) points out that the "THC" currently available "on the street" is rarely tetrahydrocannabinol, but rather phencyclidine, mescaline or LSD.

Shorthand expressions are occasionally coined with tongue in cheek, as when $T7$ is used as an abbreviation for a laboratory determination based on measurement of $T3$ (tri-iodothyronine) and $T4$ (thyroxine). Some are frankly whimsical or jocular, like *TLC = tender, loving care* and *3-H enema = high, hot and hell of a lot.*

An acronym is a word made up of the first letters of a set of other words, like *N*orth *A*tlantic *T*reaty *O*rganization and *S*elf-*C*ontained *U*nderwater *B*reathing *A*pparatus. If physicians pronounced *BUN* "bun" (which they never under any circumstances do) it would be an acronym. On the other hand, BSP could never become one because it cannot be pronounced as a word. For the same reason *DIVP = dilute intravenous Pitocin* is disqualified as an acronym, whereas *DING = drip infusion nephrotomogram* was no doubt planned as one from the beginning.

Once an acronym has come into being, it can function as a stem in the formation of compound words. *Desoxyribonucleic acid,* now generally abbreviated *DNA,* was formerly known as *DORN,* and a streptococcal enzyme that breaks down this substance was thus named *streptodornase.*

When the *ECHO = enteric cytopathogenic human orphan* virus was first isolated, it was believed not to cause any disease; hence the fanciful epithet *orphan. IMViC* is a well-known acronym for *indole–methyl red–Voges-Proskauer–citrate,* representing the set of four tests used to detect fecal contamination of water. *REM* sleep is that phase of sleep characterized by *rapid eye movements.* Almost but not quite an acronym is *arbovirus* (for *arthropod-borne virus*).

Though acronyms are not especially numerous in medical terminology, students of medicine have traditionally made use of a vast number of mnemonics, many of them unprintable, based upon a similar principle. The word *insular,* for instance, contains clues to the diagnostic features of multiple sclerosis: *i*ntention tremor, *n*ystagmus, *s*canning speech, *u*rinary difficulties and *l*oss of *a*bdominal *r*eflexes.

Most physicians have scores of these memory aids tucked away in the recesses of their minds, though as the things themselves become part of daily thought, the methods used to remember them grow obsolete and are themselves nearly forgotten. A slightly different sort of mnemonic is that exemplified in the jingle for recalling, in sequence, the names of the twelve cranial nerves:

> "On old Olympus' towering tops,
> A fop and glutton vended some hops."

An alternate last line, which makes no more sense and does not even rhyme, is

"A Finn and German vaulted some hedges."

Besides abbreviations, another form of shorthand speech and writing is the arbitrarily chosen letter or number symbol. Arabic numerals are often employed in a scale running from 1 to 4 (or 1-plus to 4-plus), according to which anything from prostatic enlargement to glycosuria can be roughly graded. Other uses of Arabic numerals include the typing of bacterial and viral strains and the gauges of catheters, dilators and suture materials.

Roman numerals are employed even more extensively, as in the grading of cardiac murmurs (two scales) and of hypertensive changes in the retina, and in distinguishing the clotting factors and the phenotypes of hyperlipidemia. They are also used as numerals in their own right in prescriptions and drug orders.

Arbitrary letter symbols are also popular. Roman letters are used to designate vitamins, blood types and groups of hemolytic streptococci. Though most letter symbols are drawn from the first part of the alphabet, exceptions include the P, Q, R, S and T waves of the electrocardiogram, X and Y chromosomes and x rays. Some expressions containing letters refer to the shapes of those letters, as in L-forms and Z-plasty.

Modern science has made extensive use of the Greek alphabet. Greek letters are applied to everything from stars *(alpha Centauri)* to radioactive emissions *(gamma irradiation)*. The mathematicians, having exhausted both the Roman and the Greek alphabets, have actually started on the Hebrew. In chemistry, Greek letters denote ring positions of cyclic compounds; in pharmacology we speak of *alpha* and *beta* adrenergic receptors; in microbiology, of *alpha* and *beta* hemolysis. Greek letters are used also to designate the secretory cells of the pancreatic islets, the rhythms of the electroencephalogram, and serum components like lipoproteins and globulins that are separated by electrophoresis.

A few symbols that are neither letters nor numerals have found their way into medical shorthand. The popular symbols for *male* and *female* are adapted from ancient astrological marks, the former representing the arrow of Mars and the latter the mirror of Venus. In modern stylized representations, the string-slot of the arrow is usually blown up into a huge circle the same size as the plate of the mirror, while the shaft of the arrow, which is the essential part of the symbol, shrinks to the size of the handle of the mirror. Physicians often use plain vertical arrows in informal notes to indicate increases and decreases or movements up and down, and horizontal arrows to denote cause-and-effect relationships on the analogy of their use in chemical equations.

𝔗𝔯𝔞𝔡𝔢 𝔑𝔞𝔪𝔢𝔰

> *The American advertiser is also a very diligent manufacturer of wholly new terms, and many of his coinages . . . have come into general acceptance as common nouns.*
>
> H. L. Mencken
> *The American Language (2)*

Trade names comprise a significant part of the terminology of medicine, as they do of the vernacular. Some, like *Bovie* and *Bird,* are simply manufacturers' names that have come to stand for certain products or appliances, as do the terms *Cadillac* and *Leica.* Others are made-up words, which run the gamut between coinages from Greek *(Elastoplast)* and variations on English words *(Stockinette).*

Just as the public has taken up some prominent trade names like *Frigidaire* and *Kleenex* and applied them generically to all similar products, so the medical profession often absorbs a trade name into its vocabulary and, eventually forgetting its origin, drops the capital letter. *Vaseline* is Chesebrough's trade name for petrolatum, introduced in 1872. Supposedly the term is a compound of German *Wasser=water,* Greek *elaion=oil* and the suffix *–ine. Kerlix, Telfa, Adaptic, Tubegauz* and, of course, *Band-Aid* are all trade names for dressing materials. *Hyfrecator* is The Burdick Company's registered trademark for its *hi*gh *f*requency electrodesic*cator.*

Perhaps the majority of trade names that physicians use are patented drug names. The naming of new drugs poses a continuing challenge to pharmaceutical manufacturers and to the medical profession, for each drug name must be different enough from all others to minimize the risk of confusion in speech and writing. The ideal name is also relatively short, easy to spell and pronounce, and associated in some way with the composition or action of the drug.

The systematization of generic (nonproprietary) drug names in recent years has been a noteworthy achievement. Though terms like *edetate* and *pamoate* draw chuckles from professional chemists, they are

2. Mencken HL: THE AMERICAN LANGUAGE. Copyright held by Alfred A. Knopf, Inc., New York, p214

at least easier for physicians to remember and write than *ethyl-enediaminetetraacetate* or *4, 4'-methylenbis (3-hydroxy-2-naphthoate)*. The United States Adopted Names (USAN) Council was formed in 1964 to adopt appropriate generic names for all new drugs developed in the United States. Sponsored jointly by the American Medical Association, the American Pharmaceutical Association and the United States Pharmacopoeial Convention, Inc., the Council works with pharmaceutical manufacturers in the selection of meaningful and distinctive names for new drugs, and cooperates with other national and international agencies toward a maximum degree of standardization in generic naming of drugs. (3).

The brand names chosen for drugs, though subject to approval by the Federal Food and Drug Administration, are of course invented by the manufacturers. So difficult has it become to select new drug names that will satisfy all the other requirements, and will also look good on a label and sound melodious to the ear, that drug manufacturers have resorted to mechanical fabrication of names. Hundreds of prefixes, suffixes and stems are fed into a computer and matched at random. In a printout of several thousand specimens, only a handful may be worthy of consideration; some must be rejected because they are too much like existing names, others because they are misleading, ludicrous, or simply ugly.

Drug manufacturers go to great lengths to ensure that names chosen for new drugs will be pleasing to the ear and easily remembered. In one study, physicians chosen at random were sent a list of ten proposed drug names and asked to indicate which ones they found pleasant-sounding and what they thought might be the nature and purpose of each. A few weeks later, to their surprise, they received a second letter asking how many of the names in the list they could remember; this, of course, was the real point of the study.

Brand names of drugs range from the ingenious to the bizarre. Some are based, straightforwardly enough, on therapeutic action: *Diuril,* a diuretic; *Apresoline,* an antihypertensive; *Lomotil,* a drug to reduce intestinal motility. The physician is usually on safe ground if he concludes that a drug whose name ends in *–ase* is an enzyme or that a *–mycin* or a *–myxin* is an antibiotic. The syllables *cort, cill, bel* and *barb* almost invariably point, respectively, to an adrenal cortical hormone, a penicillin, a belladonna alkaloid, and a barbiturate.

At times the effort to keep drugs of like kind together results in

3. The "Guiding Principles for USAN" were published in JAMA 213:608, 1970; see also "The USAN Nomenclature System," JAMA 232:294, 1975

the coinage of misleading names. *Cocaine* (from *coca,* the plant source, and *–ine,* the alkaloid suffix) was the first local anesthetic used in modern surgery. When a synthetic drug was developed that had less serious side-effects, it was called *procaine* (from Latin *pro=for* and *–caine,* a fragment arbitrarily chopped off *cocaine*) and first marketed as *Novocain* (from Latin *novus=new*). Since then most newly developed local anesthetic drugs have been called *–caines* whether they are chemically related to the parent drug or not.

Sometimes a brand name is a phonetic spelling of the generic name or part of it *(Sudafed=pseudoephedrine; Ascodeen=aspirin with codeine),* or even of letters *(Kay-Ciel=KCl, potassium chloride);* others represent simplifications of cumbersome terms *(Carfusin=carbol fuchsin)* or eponyms *(Vlem-Dome=Vleminckx' solution).* Many are built up of other trade names *(Combid=Compazine* and *Darbid; Ser-Ap-Es=Serpasil, Apresoline* and *Esidrix).*

A few are true acronyms: *DOPA=dihydroxyphenylalanine; Capla=* *c*entrally *a*cting *p*ressure-*l*owering *a*gent; *Ansolysen,* a ganglionic blocking agent, from *a*utonomic *n*ervous *s*ystem and Greek *lysis=loosening.* The coumarin derivative *warfarin,* first marketed as a rodenticide, was not so called because man's effort to control the rat population is a never-ending warfare, but after the *W*isconsin *A*lumni *R*esearch *F*oundation and the last four letters of the chemical name. Later, when the chemical was released for use as an anticoagulant in human medicine, one brand, *Panwarfin,* preserved the acronymic reference to the original developers. *Premarin* is built up from *pr*egnant *mar*es' ur*ine,* which indicates the source of the drug.

Among oddities may be mentioned *Amen, Miltown, Marplan* and *Letter,* which do not sound like drug names at all and for that reason are probably much easier to remember. A levo-rotatory isomer of *Darvon* (dextro-propoxyphene) bears the mirror-image name *Novrad.* Many brand names contain references to the manufacturer's name: *Robitussin* and *Robinul,* made by A. H. Robins; *Wyanoids* and *Wycillin,* by Wyeth; *Talwin* by Winthrop. Smith, Kline and French markets a line of drugs beginning with a phonetic spelling of *S, K: Eskatrol, Eskabarb.*

The pronunciation of drug names has a way of following the laws of popular speech instead of the wishes of the manufacturer. *Xylocaine* was meant to be accented on the second syllable, to emphasize that it is a *local* anesthetic, but it is almost never so pronounced. *Banthine* and *Pro-Banthine* are supposed to rhyme with *wine,* but seldom do. There is no uniformity whatever in the pronunciation of *Enovid, Lomotil* and *Valium.*

Spelling, too, is sometimes erratic. *Demerol* turns up in an astonishing variety of forms. *Nembutal* often loses its *m*, *Dulcolax* its first *l*, *Carbrital* its second *r*; pHisoHex and NTZ are seldom given the correct apportionment of large and small capital letters in handwritten orders and records. Even generic names are subject to frequent distortion: witness *meprobromate*, often heard for *meprobamate*, and *amyl nitrate*, for *nitrite*. Webster lists five alternative pronunciations for *reserpine*.

6

slang, jargon, and gibberish

Medicalese I

That night he started *putting out* some *red stuff*
through his *Foley*. The *clerk* happened to be *on the
floor* and *did a urine on* him, and it was *loaded* with
red cells. We got the *GU boys* to *scope* him . . .
                                    —*Heard at Grand Rounds*

The special language of a trade or profession can be divided into
technical terminology and argot. We have dealt hitherto with the formal language of medicine, as it is codified in medical dictionaries and
employed in textbooks and printed material generally. We turn now to
a consideration of those informal, unconventional, and unorthodox
usages peculiar to the spoken idiom of medicine, which may be designated as medical argot, medical slang, or simply medicalese.

It is easier to recognize slang than to define it, but perhaps its most
essential trait is simply its unconventionality, its inappropriateness in a
formal letter or an interview between relative strangers, its absence
from the dictionary. Not that there is necessarily anything incorrect,
improper or degrading about argot. We all use, or at least understand,
argots of various kinds. Every trade, every sport, and indeed every
plane and species of human endeavor has its own special language, from
television quiz shows *(mystery guest, consolation prize)* to kidnapping *(ran-
som note, drop)*. It is not even accurate to say that whereas all formal
medical terminology is fit to print, medical argot is not, for the only
writers of medical literature who consistently avoid using argot are
those who are not physicians, and the result of their diffidence and
ignorance is a loss in intelligibility rather than a gain. Of the informal
usages catalogued in the following pages, the great majority contribute

more to the succinctness and vigor of medical language than they take away from its purity and elegance; otherwise they would probably never have come into being.

Like nearly all argots, medicalese is a dynamic and rapidly evolving medium, with regional peculiarities and shifting conventions. Many slang expressions prove ephemeral: *hypo = hypodermic injection* and *psycho = psychotic*, after enjoying a certain vogue in medicalese and even drifting into the vernacular, are now nearly extinct. Others, despite frequent splenetic outbursts from editors of medical journals, become legitimized by long usage and are assumed into the conventional language of medicine: *leucocytosis with a left shift, a high index of suspicion.*

Virtually every slang expression is either a metaphor *(gourd = cranium)*, a neologism *(crock [1] = hypochondriac)*, or an altered form of a conventional word *(sed rate = sedimentation rate, orthopod = orthopedist)*. To a great extent medicalese consists of common English words applied in special ways. The preposition *on,* for example, has acquired the meaning *under treatment with,* as in "Let's put him on digitalis." This is probably an outgrowth of a venerable usage in the vernacular *(on dope, on the sauce)*. In medicalese, though, it is often extended to modes of treatment other than drugs ("He was put on postural drainage") and to diagnostic procedures ("He was put on strained urines"). Patients may be *put, placed, tried, started* or even *begun* on all of these things. The opposite idea is expressed, logically enough, by *off:* "I took him off gold and put him on iron." *On* also means *about* or *in the case of,* as "We did a count on her" or "We may have to go in on him yet tonight." Still another sense of this word is exemplified in "On auscultation a pericardial friction rub was heard" and "On section the liver was hyperemic." (Contrast *at laparatomy, at autopsy.*) Finally, *on* is of course a well-established abbreviation for *on duty* in medicine as in many other fields.

To run appears in several specialized expressions, where it can mean *to perform a diagnostic test* ("We ran serial blood cultures") or *to display a symptom or sign* ("He was running three- and four-plus albumins"). *To have* enters into an even wider variety of idioms, perhaps most of them parallel to expressions in the general language. A patient can *have* a symptom (chills), a sign (crepitant rales), a disease (pneumonia), a diagnostic procedure (sputum smear), a laboratory finding (gram-positive diplococci), a drug (penicillin), a therapeutic procedure (bronchoscopy), a surgical operation (segmental resection) and an uneventful recovery. A patient can even *have* something that he does not have: "She had absent breath sounds at the left base posteriorly."

1. Or is this a corruption of *chronic,* or *crank,* or German *krank = sick?*

In order to *have* all these things, patients must first *get* them. In a discussion of a given disease among a group of medical men one often hears expressions like "They [*i.e.,* patients afflicted with this disease] get a microcytic, hypochromic anemia" and "Can't they sometimes get a relative lymphocytosis?" *Get* also means *to order or perform a test* ("I got a bilirubin"), *to be treated with* ("He was getting chlorpromazine") or *to become* ("He was getting jaundiced").

To pass means *to discharge or expel some material or substance from a natural or other orifice,* as blood in the urine, stones in the bile, or mucus in the stool. *To spill* ("She's spilling sugar and acetone") is used only for substances excreted abnormally in the urine.

Besides its rather straightforward though metaphorical use to mean that an unconscious patient is "coming to," the verb *respond* may be applied to a disease that improves with treatment: "Anginal pain responded to nitroglycerine." Both patients and diseases may also be said to *present:* "The patient presented with sudden complete loss of vision in the right eye"; "Multiple sclerosis may present as acute urinary retention."

A *study* is any diagnostic procedure ("radiographic studies of the colon," "liver function studies"), but *work* usually implies clinical laboratory tests, as exemplified in the curiously elliptic *fasting blood work.* Regrettably, many a *workup=thorough diagnostic evaluation* consists largely of laboratory *work.*

The figurative use of *read* is well established in the vernacular: "Let's take a reading," "Do you read me?" Physicians *read* x rays, electrocardiograms, electroencephalograms, thermometers, and even skin tests. *To monitor* is *to maintain surveillance over a natural or abnormal state or process by frequent or continuous collection of data. To see* a patient is *to interview, examine* and/or *treat* him; *to follow* him is to continue to *see* him at intervals. *To scrub on a case,* or simply *to scrub,* means to take an active part in a surgical procedure.

An intravenous infusion of fluid has long been known as a *drip* because of the drip-chamber method of noting flow rate. In recent years the rapid injection of the entire contents of a syringe directly into a vein has come to be known as a *push.* It may also be called an *IV bolus,* by analogy with the old-fashioned method of making up a dose of bad-tasting medicine in a large wad of dough or molasses. This dosage form, still much used in veterinary medicine, was called a *bolus* from Greek *bolos=a clod of earth.* Bottles of intravenous solution connected in tandem are said to be *piggybacked.* (*Tandem* is itself an old slang word, borrowed by schoolboys from Latin. The classical sense of the word is *finally,* and its application to a two-seated bicycle is a punning allusion to the linear disposition of the riders: "at length.")

The argot of medicine includes a number of usages that many physicians probably do not regard as unconventional, even though they vary considerably from formal or dictionary applications of the words used. Some of these usages, like the examples cited in foregoing paragraphs, involve ordinary English words: acute hepatic *insult*, a *generous* biopsy, to *discourage* keloid formation, diabetes *intractable* to oral *agents*, peptic ulcer *refractory* to conservative *management*, an *episode* of hypoglycemia, *documented* pancreatitis, a pulmonary *cripple*, *classical* migraine, lymphocytes are *elevated*. *Secondary to* now invariably means not merely *following after* but *caused by*.

In many other instances technical words that have a strict meaning in the dictionary are used in much broader senses in daily speech and even sometimes in formal writing: *chronic* anticonvulsant therapy, the synovial fluid was *noninflammatory*, the patient was *operated* for cholelithiasis, she looks *toxic*. Any abnormality whatever may be called a *lesion* ("the biochemical lesion of gout") and any disorder in which objective evidence of a lesion is lacking may be designated as *functional* (2).

Forming an extensive class of words in this category are those ending in *–logy*. People in general seem to have an irresistible impulse to apply these words not to the fields of study that they denote, but to the objects of study. *Psychology* has been employed with increasing latitude since the late nineteenth century, and *ecology* is nowadays suffering the same kind of abuse. The explanation of this tendency may lie in the example of a few such words (*analogy, eulogy, tetralogy*) that do not refer to the study of anything, but is more likely to be found in the succinctness that can be achieved by using a *–logy* word: "This symptomatology persisted despite absence of demonstrable pathology, and only when a routine serology was reported as strongly reactive did the etiology become obvious." Each of the *–logy* terms in this sentence conveys an idea that would take two to four words to express otherwise.

The long-established *pathologic fracture* derives its significance from the notion that there can be *pathology* in a bone. The application of the term *pathology* to diseases and abnormalities of every description has begun at last to generate a mild reaction. Some physicians, guiltily uneasy about saying things like "There was no pathology in the liver," have actually substituted the extraordinary neologism *pathosis*. It is bad enough to misapply an existing word, but it is even worse to fabricate

2. This latter word has acquired strange connotations in other fields than medicine. In architecture and interior decorating many consider it synonymous with *ugly!*

a new one when we already have *disease, abnormality, disturbance, irregularity* and many other more suitable expressions. Sometimes a *–logy* word seems to be chosen simply because it sounds more scientific, as when *morphology* is substituted for *shape.*

Names of sciences that do not end in *–logy* are also frequently applied to the subject matter in a broad fashion: "an anatomic abnormality," "a flaw in iron chemistry." A similar usage is *morbidity* in the extremely vague sense of *incidence, severity or duration of illness.*

If many of these usages seem to hover between argot and conventional language, other forms of medicalese quite plainly represent a deliberate retreat from formal technical terminology, as when a severed blood vessel is called a *bleeder* (or *spurter* or *gusher*) or a contaminated instrument is referred to as *dirty,* a blood culture is said to be *cooking* or *Mycobacterium tuberculosis* is called the *red bug* or *red snapper* (allusions to its appearance in a smear stained by the acid-fast method).

Some informal locutions are particularly vigorous (*"slap* a PPD on him," "he *blew out* an aneurysm," "she's been *throwing* PVCs," "they *reamed out* his left carotid three years ago"), even brutal ("I think it's time to *yank* his *gizzard,"* "he needs a dose of *cold steel* [=*surgery*]," "we'll have to *crack her squash* [=*perform craniotomy*]."

Another large class of medicalese comprises syncopated, abbreviated or elliptical expressions. Many of these are one-word technical terms of which part has been dropped: [*electro*]*lytes,* [*electrocardio*]*gram, multip*[*ara*], *osteo*[*myelitis*], *staph*[*ylococcus*], *strep*[*tococcus*]. *Scope* is applied as both noun and verb to virtually every kind of 'scope except the stethoscope. Though *aortic regurge*=*regurgitation* and *rehab*=*rehabilitation* are still considered a bit vulgar, *consult*=*consultation, assist*=*assistance at surgery* and *hemostat*=*hemostatic forceps* are now quite generally accepted.

Even more numerous are expressions in which only part of a phrase is retained for the whole: *white* [*blood cell*] *count, differential* [*white blood cell count*] or [*diagnosis*], [*adrenal cortical*] *steroid,* [*x-ray examination of the*] *upper GI* [*tract*], *post* [*mortem examination*]. *Coronary,* for *coronary artery thrombosis,* has been abandoned by the medical profession in favor of [*myocardial*] *infarct,* and is now a lay term. In many of these elliptic expressions it seems that the part retained is the least important or meaningful of all, as when a gynecologist speaks of the *portio* [*vaginalis of the cervix*] or a thoracic surgeon of a *pectus* [*excavatum*]. We also hear *cor pulmonale* spoken of as simply *cor,* and the usual adjectival form of *vena cava* is plain *caval.* As these examples suggest, this sort of truncation is especially common with non-English phrases. It also occurs with taxonomic terms for microorganisms; the frequent use of *coli* for *Bacillus* (later *Escherichia*) *coli* led to the formation, early in this century, of the mongrel adjective *coliform,* which survives to this day. Another irregularity of this kind that has been ratified by usage is the conversion of the active participle *alternans* (as in *pulsus alternans*) into a substantive: *electrical alternans.*

The process of ellipsis goes a step further when a complex idea is compressed into a two-word phrase or compound such as may well appear to the uninitiated to mean something quite different. (Plain English is full of such expressions; imagine a foreigner with a pocket dictionary trying to decipher *quarter horse, flea collar* or *baby-sitter.*) Examples of this type of syncopation in medicalese are *acute abdomen* (also known as a *red-hot belly*), *acute facility, febrile agglutinins, extrapyramidal signs, liver panel, lordotic films* and *patient days.* The newly-named *Drug Enforcement Administration* enforces not drugs but laws pertaining to them. Yet another instance is *mad doctor,* which formerly meant a physician specializing in the treatment of mental illness, though in the modern horror film and Gothic novel it generally has a more literal significance.

The epithets that physicians apply to their patients may sometimes seem to indicate a certain lack of compassion or humanity, but the technical language is limited in terms for patients. We have words like *cretin, diabetic* and *cirrhotic,* but what do you call a person who has cancer or coronary artery disease, or who has suffered a stroke or been shot? The usual recourse is to say that the patient *"is* a lymphosarcoma of the stomach,"* though occasionally expressions like *a stroker* or *a GI bleeder* are used. *Aphake* and *myope* are almost indispensable terms in ophthalmology, where they are no longer considered slang.

Though they readily stretch the meanings of words, physicians show little imagination or initiative in the fabrication of new words in medicalese. Exceptions are *retrospectoscope,* a mythical instrument with which the pathologist is reputed to achieve 20/20 hindsight in identifying the errors and omissions of the clinician, and the acronymic *Gok's disease* (God only knows).

Not all medicalese has arisen within the medical profession. As physicians have come into contact with representatives of commerce, government, and technology they have borrowed and adapted words from the argots of these fields. The language of business has contributed several expressions that seem particularly out of place in medicine. *Counterproductive* may be appropriate when applied to something done in a factory, but hardly when said of what is done in a hospital or a physician's office. Terms like *health industry, health services consumer, health maintenance organization* and *delivery of care* seem to degrade the practice of medicine from a professional activity to a commercial enterprise or, worse, a purely mechanical process.

However inappropriate these expressions may seem when transplanted into the language of medicine, the workaday argot of the businessman is in general a terse and serviceable idiom. When, for example, he writes a memorandum beginning "per our telecon re . . ." instead of "as we discussed in our telephone conversation about . . ." he is saving time and space with no sacrifice of intelligibility.

Very different is that extraordinary jargon known to professional writers as *gobbledygook,* which is employed in the drafting of legislation, in judicial opinions and technical publications, and in correspondence by government officials and civil servants. Here is a verbatim quotation from a personal letter now lying on my desk: "It would be desirable to determine his baseline profile relative to these materials prior to active participation in routine procedures in which they will be handled." This sentence of gobbledygook contains just twice as many words as the English translation: "We should determine his baseline levels of these materials before he handles them."

Gobbledygook is characterized by studied imprecision, unrestrained verbosity and an implicit denial of human involvement in anything. For straightforward English expressions, gobbledygook substitutes phrases beginning *in terms of, insofar as, on the basis of, from the standpoint of.* Human beings, when mentioned at all, are disguised under such cumbersome terms as *the above-captioned* and *the undersigned.* More often the actors remain altogether behind the scenes, and by heavy reliance on the passive voice, and liberal and shameless use of dangling modifiers, the writer contrives to get things done without them.

Not only does gobbledygook seem more like a species of mental illness than a mode of speech and writing, but it is an alarmingly contagious disorder. It is a matter of common observation that a person whose occupation obliges him to read and write letters and documents in gobbledygook eventually gets into the habit of speaking it as well. Moreover, many members of the medical profession show an unseemly predilection for this tangled and noncommittal gibberish.

Utilization, being a way of saying *use* in five syllables, delights the heart of the gobbledygook addict. *Summarization* (for *summary*) and *cauterization* (for *cautery*) belong to the same disreputable family. Modern medical writing is often encumbered with snatches of gobbledygook, as when we read that something happened *on a daily basis* instead of *daily,* or was done *at weekly intervals* instead of *weekly,* or that a rash was *pruritic in nature* instead of simply *pruritic.* Brief and pithy

English words are scrapped in favor of long-winded and often nebulous phrases, so that *neck* becomes *cervical region* and *bones* masquerade as *osseous structures.*

From computer technology medicine has borrowed expressions like *feedback, input* and *software.* A number of other words, such as *marginal, protocol* and *profile,* have penetrated medical slang from related fields. Though a few of these expressions provide convenient and succinct ways of saying things (lipid *profile,* broad-*spectrum* antibiotic), many of them lose their specific meanings when they venture beyond the disciplines to which they are relevant, and degenerate into mere jargon.

Some, for example, become non-words, useful chiefly in concealing the speaker's or writer's ignorance, confusion or laziness: *scope, factor, element, orientation, parameter.* Others contaminate everyday English as well as professional speech and writing with an unsavory taint of technicalese: an *indepth* answer, *at this point in time,* and the ubiquitous and usually meaningless *as such.* If the mathematical term *plus* continues to gain ground as a substitute in polite speech for *and* ("My nose is running plus it hurts when I swallow"), the English language may soon become the first in history to have two exactly synonymous versions of this very basic word.

Some borrowings were slang even before medicine acquired them. A *red herring* in law and politics is a false trail deliberately laid by an opponent. This is a metaphor drawn from fox-hunting, and refers to the fact that if a red (*i.e.,* smoked) herring is drawn across the trail, the hounds will go off on the false scent. The diagnostic red herrings that physicians have to deal with are usually fortuitous, though the phrase may first have become popular in medicine in conjunction with the deliberately tortuous clinicopathologic conference "protocol."

At least a century before the advent of aerial photography, architects and landscapers began calling a surface map or the plan of a large area a *bird's-eye view.* The self-evident significance of the phrase is completely lost in expressions like "a bird's-eye view of renal function." *No man's land* once meant literally a strip of unclaimed waste ground between adjacent kingdoms, but in the era of trench warfare it was applied to the zone between the trenches of opposing armies. Modern surgery uses the expression for structures or regions of the human body where certain procedures are inadvisable or impossible.

There are two highly objectionable classes of usage in medicalese, both of them characteristic of written or dictated clinical records. One consists of words and phrases that generally bear testimony to a certain bias or lack of intellectual honesty. For example, reference to the *unex-*

plained hostility of the patient is often merely a means of disguising the physician's own hostility or insecurity. The physician may unjustly describe as *uncooperative* a patient who despite the most heroic efforts is unable to produce a specimen of sputum. The ever-recurring note that the patient is a *poor historian* can often be attributed to a physician who was too tired or too rushed to take a good history from a deaf or confused patient.

The other category of undesirable language in medical record-keeping is the use of the hedging modifier. A radiologist interprets spine films of two patients and dictates identical descriptions of his findings. Why, then, is his conclusion for the first patient "Normal dorsal and lumbar spine" and for the second, "Findings would suggest an essentially normal dorsal and lumbar spine at this time?"

Would and *suggest* rob the second report of conviction; *essentially* and *at this time* hint at exceptions to *normal.* Here is what the radiologist is really saying: "The patient has clinical signs of organic disease of the spine; something abnormal ought to be visible on these films, but I see nothing. Another radiologist, reviewing these films and comparing them with later ones, may see incipient changes here that I have overlooked. A report of absolute normalcy may seem to justify omission of further diagnostic studies, and may later seem to reflect on my abilities, yet I cannot identify the slightest variation from normal on these films."

A first-year internal medicine resident writes in an admitting note: "Heart: 116, regular, no heave or thrill, no murmur, no definite gallop rhythm . . . no true peripheral edema . . ." What is a *definite* gallop rhythm? What is *true* edema? If the patient has *no* gallop rhythm and *no* edema, why not simply say so?

Here is what the note really means: "I think the patient is in congestive heart failure. My staff man will expect me to have looked for a gallop rhythm and peripheral edema. I have done so, and found neither, but tomorrow morning on rounds he will probably find both. By inserting these hedging modifiers, *definite* and *real,* I leave myself a loophole: if the abnormal signs are present in the opinion of the staff man, my choice of expressions may be interpreted to mean that I felt these findings were 'borderline.' If not, my statements can stand at face value."

𝔐𝔢𝔡𝔦𝔠𝔞𝔩𝔢𝔰𝔢 II

Psychologists and sociologists, economists and biologists, mathematicians and statisticians, neurologists and anthropologists have evolved such subtle and elaborate technical languages, or metalanguages as we may perhaps call them, that they stand in serious danger of forgetting how to speak simply and plainly to others who happen to find themselves outside their own peculiar circle. These specialists are indeed the victims of a kind of endemic semiliteracy, which, in its more acute stages, may result in linguistic paralysis and aphasia.

Simeon Potter
Modern Linguistics (3)

The physician who spends much of his time in direct contact with adult patients usually develops a hybrid jargon for use in discussing diagnoses and treatments with them. For example, he may refer to a diuretic injection as a *water shot,* gastroenteritis as *stomach flu,* and a vaginal examination as an *internal.*

In most such instances, a slight sacrifice of scientific accuracy is justified by the improvement in intelligibility. Even when physicians pick up such wholly erroneous lay usages as *pill* (strictly speaking, always spherical) for anything from lozenges to capsules, or *nauseous* (which means *sickening*) in the sense of *nauseated,* the result is most often smoother communication. Indeed, there are times when insistence on precise terminology is pointless, even undesirable. The physician who makes the mistake of mentioning *neurodermatitis* to an educated patient may encounter a storm of recrimination as the patient erroneously interprets the word to mean *skin trouble due to nervousness.*

Some physicians display a rigid incapacity for avoiding technical terms when speaking to patients. It is as though their thoughts were so firmly wedded to the technical language of medicine that they cannot "think lay." A "patient flyer" (4) approved by the Food and Drug Administration for inclusion in packages of intrauterine devices contains this sentence: "If [you become pregnant and] the IUD is not removed, you should know that there is an increased risk of an infected abortion occurring when the pregnancy is allowed to continue." Quite apart from its grammatical irregularities, which do not obscure its meaning, this sentence is objectionable because its use of the word *abortion* is likely to confuse a majority of lay readers. Though abortion originally denoted miscarriage and only later acquired the meaning of

3. Potter S: MODERN LINGUISTICS. London, Andre Deutsch, Ltd., 1967
4. FDA Drug Bulletin, December, 1974

an active and deliberate interruption of pregnancy, this latter meaning is virtually the only one popularly recognized. It makes no difference that the IUD is in fact an abortifacient device; the phrase "infected abortion occurring when the pregnancy is allowed to continue" is bound to be sheer doubletalk to the average lay reader.

An even more remarkable instance of unduly technical language in printed material intended for the lay reader is this inscription on the package of a pediculocide: "If accidental ingestion occurs, prompt institution of gastric lavage will rid the body of large amounts of the toxicant. However, since oils favor absorption, saline cathartics for intestinal evacuation should be given rather than oil laxatives . . . If irritation or sensitization occurs, discontinue the product and consult physician." The last sentence is included merely to convince the justly incredulous reader that this masterpiece of obnubilation is indeed meant for nonprofessional eyes. Does the layman know how to "institute" gastric lavage? Does he know a saline cathartic from a duodenal diverticulum? Does he appreciate the distinction between irritation and sensitization? Even a dictionary may not help him much, for *toxicant* appears in none that I have seen except THE OXFORD ENGLISH DICTIONARY and the unabridged WEBSTER, neither of which is likely to grace the shelves of anyone who cannot figure out the meaning of the word for himself.

The adoption of lay expressions does not, of course, automatically guarantee greater intelligibility. It is true that *spinal tap* is not only more meaningful and less painful-sounding to the patient than *lumbar puncture,* but actually a little more accurate, and that *hardening of the arteries* is a literal rendering of *arteriosclerosis* into plain English. But it seems doubtful that *the walls of the heart, the lining of the chest* or *the neck of the womb* conveys any more information to the anatomically unsophisticated than *myocardium, pleura* or *cervix.*

There are some cases in which the uncritical adoption of a surrogate expression for a more abstruse term may carry the potential of actual harm to the patient. Consider the careless way in which both patients and physicians throw around the expression *kidney infection.* The difference between cystitis and pyelonephritis is more than a verbal quibble, but all too often *kidney infection* is used as a generic term for both. *Colitis* is a frequent misnomer for disturbances of colonic function without organic disease.

Some physicians have a regrettable habit of inventing, or at least misapplying, terms to cover their inability to arrive at a diagnosis. There must be several million people in this country who have been told by physicians that they have *low blood pressure,* a condition unknown to writers of textbooks of medicine. Informing a patient that his joint pains are due to *arthralgia* or diagnosing a sore throat as *pharyngitis* is playing at word games, not practicing medicine. One is reminded of Kant's observation that physicians think they have done a great deal for the patient when they have given his disease a name.

No doubt we are all guilty from time to time of evading unpleasant issues by using euphemisms like *growth* for *malignancy,* or noncommittal words like *weight* for *obesity* or *problem* for *alcoholism.* But if it is true that we ought to avoid, when possible, such emotionally-charged words as *cancer, epilepsy, underdeveloped* and *senile,* we should also make it a rule to avoid substitute terms that are nebulous *(the beginnings of an ulcer),* elusive *(a blood condition)* or so inaccurate that they actually mean something else *(excess acid in the system; heart spasms).*

𝔐𝔢𝔡𝔦𝔠𝔞𝔩𝔢𝔰𝔢 𝔏𝔏𝔏

Subtle: Infuse vinegar,
To draw his volatile substance and his tincture:
And let the water in glass E be filt'red,
And put into the gripe's egg. Lute him well;
And leave him closed *in balneo.*
Face: [*within*]   I will, sir.
Surly: What a brave language here is! Next to canting.

Ben Jonson
The Alchemist

Besides the special jargon that physicians use when they speak to patients about technical matters, there is yet another *patois* in which doctors converse among themselves about these matters when they must do so in the presence of the patient. The former idiom is intended to make complex ideas intelligible, the latter to make simple ideas opaque. Most clinical teaching is done in the patient's presence (and often within earshot of several of his ward-mates). Though he may not understand much of what he hears, he can hardly help recognizing and making some sense out of references to unwelcome diagnoses and impending catastrophes. Hence it is customary to couch embarrassing or disagreeable subjects in a kind of doubletalk that only another medical man is expected to understand.

For instance, one does not speak of a tentative diagnosis of *syphilis* before the patient; one uses the archaic *lues.* If the patient's *heart* is his weak spot, we talk of his *cor;* if we think he has something wrong with his *liver,* we discuss his *hepar.* If, further, we attribute that liver trouble to the chronic abuse of alcohol, we may refer to *ethanolism* or *chronic overexposure to EtOH.* If we fear that the patient has a malignancy, we discuss a *neoplasm* or a *space-occupying* (or *mitotic* [5]) *lesion. Blood* is called *hemoglobin, heme, red cells, erythrocytes, RBCs.*

If the patient's death seems imminent, it may be suggested that the exact nature of his trouble will presently be elucidated by Dr. MacTavish (or Schultz, or Paglioni, or whoever is the hospital pathologist). A patient whose complaints seem largely imaginary, or at least unrelated to any organic disease, is said to have a *supratentorial problem.* Occasionally one hears that such a patient has a *high serum porcelain level,* an allusion to the slang term *crock.* A patient whose intelligence seems limited is spoken of as having *Betz cell atrophy,* though Betz cells are motor neurons and have nothing to do with intelligence. Some speakers even plunge further into absurdity and talk of *Betz cell anemia.*

If the patient is obese, the fact is evident to all observers, and yet sometimes the matter must be discussed at the bedside. We then refer to his *panniculus* or his *excess of signet ring cells.*

Since physicians at a teaching center customarily speak of private medical practitioners and other referring physicians as though they were incompetent, irresponsible and slightly crooked, they are a little reluctant to refer to the patient's family doctor by name. Accordingly, he becomes the *PMD* or *LMD (private* or *local M. D.).* In his turn, the PMD professes to deplore the fragmented and impersonal style of medicine practiced in the *ivory* (a nearly universal corruption of *ivied*) *tower.*

Doctors occasionally use expressions that seem perfectly innocent to them but that patients interpret in an altogether different way. Every medical student has heard the story about the attending physician who on ward rounds put his hand on a female patient's chest, drily remarked that he felt a *thrill,* and was rewarded with a slap in the face. What must a patient think who learns that his physicians plan to *get a liver panel on him,* or who hears himself characterized as a *possible chronic brain?*

5. The reference here is to the microscopic appearance of malignant tissue. Such tissue displays much "chromosomal activity," though the form of cell division characteristic of malignant tissue is not *mitosis,* which is normal, but rather *amitosis.*

Patientese

*The doctor contributed everything to my gall, and
gave me a subscription to strengthen my kidneys.*

—Anonymous

Physicians do not have a monopoly on the use of medical terminology. The language of medicine, with its resounding polysyllabic words and its aura of the scientific and the mysterious, has always exercised an irresistible fascination upon the lay mind. From the middle ages almost to our own day, any mountebank with a few scraps of Latin at his command was able to hoodwink the gullible into believing him a learned and skillful practitioner.

Patients themselves delight in exchanging exotic-sounding diagnoses and comparing drug names, but their inability to remember such words accurately is legendary and can be used as an argument both for and against labeling prescription packages with drug names. It is true that the patient cannot go far wrong as long as the label is in front of him. When it is not, however, his recollection of the name of the drug undergoes curious metamorphoses. A professional chemist once assured me with some heat that in 1965 another physician had treated him for a skin rash with *sulfanilamide* tablets. Patients frequently confound *grains, grams* and *milligrams;* one told me he was taking *two thousand grams* of Vitamin C daily.

The medical language of the layman, insofar as it varies from that of the physician, can be considered under the fourfold division of standard English, dialect, conscious slang and error. When we examined medical English in Chapter 2 we were concerned with English words and phrases that are used by the medical profession as part of its technical vocabulary. A great many lay expressions never find their way into the speech of physicians. Such, for instance, are *rupture* for *hernia, boil* for *abscess, hives* for *urticaria* and *shingles* for *herpes zoster.* A patient often says he has *stoved* a finger or feels a *stitch* in his side or a *crick* in his neck or that his eye is *mattering,* though these terms are not likely to get into the doctor's records. Patients customarily call any injection a *shot,* which may be qualified by an adjective that indicates the problem that the shot is supposed to prevent *(tetanus shot)* or alleviate *(pain shot),* the drug injected *(penicillin shot)* or even the location of the injection *(hip shot).*

Some common vernacular expressions are avoided by physicians because they are misleading or inaccurate: *heartburn* has nothing to do with the heart, and *hay fever* does not cause a fever. The physician may be reluctant to call herpes labialis a *cold sore* or a *fever blister* in a patient who has neither a cold nor a fever, and he may speak of *Rhus* or *urushiol* or *venenate dermatitis*, preferring to limit the meaning of *poison ivy* to the plant itself.

Standard English includes many euphemisms, such as *period = menstruation, cramps = dysmenorrhea, passage = defecation, irregularity = constipation* and *expire = die*. It also contains a host of old-fashioned terms that were once used in medicine but have now died out: *wen = sebaceous cyst, physic* or *cathartic = laxative,* and *rheumatism = any aches in joints or muscles.* Certain lay terms have been created, or at least perpetuated, by journalists and "science writers." Among these may be mentioned *birth canal, rib cage* (6) and *voice box.* Not infrequently the news media speak of a sick or injured person who is in *guarded condition.* Though I know this is simply some journalist's hashed version of "The prognosis is guarded," the expression always calls up in my mind the image of an armed policeman at the patient's bedside. We have the journalists to thank also for *miracle* and *wonder drug* and *scientific breakthrough.*

Literally hundreds of dialects are spoken within the United States, but many of them share a core of medical expressions that may be heard in almost any part of the country. A *raising* or *rising* (often pronounced *raisin'*) is any swelling on the surface of the body; it may also be called a *kernel* or a *knot.* (The *knot* often turns out to be a lymph *node,* which is cognate with *knot* and ultimately identical in meaning.) *Beal* is a variation on *boil,* and is often used in an adjectival sense *(a bealed ear).* This is an ancient dialectal word that was in use in England as early as the fourteenth century. Irritation of the skin due to friction is called *galding* ("My skin is *galded*"); these are popular corruptions of *galling* and *galled* (compare *drownding, drownded*).

Syncope is called *falling out* and diarrhea is known as *running off.* A urethral discharge is a *strain* (except when it is due to gonorrhea, in which case it is *clap* or *claps*). The primary chancre of syphilis *(blood disease; bad blood)* is a *haircut.* *Water* may mean tissue fluid, as in *water on the knee,* but more often refers to urine. *Bowels* can mean either the intestine or its discharges. *Cold* (often *col'*) refers to mucus, originally nasopharyngeal but by extension any other kind, as in "My baby is passing cold with her bowels."

Deliberately formed slang expressions for medical matters are partly the result of patients' inability to reproduce accurately the pro-

---

6. There are, according to a venerable piece of dissecting room wit, four birds in the thoracic cage: the vagoose, the esophagoose, the azygoose and the thoracic duck.

nunciation of "big" medical words, partly a reflection of their efforts to keep up their spirits in the face of suffering. Among teenagers acne pustules are commonly known as *zits,* despite the cosmetic manufacturers' insistence on the genteel euphemism *blemish.* A *shiner* is a periorbital ecchymosis, a *goose-egg* is a traumatic hematoma of the scalp.

Lay medical slang includes many of the unprintable words in the common speech connected with excretory and reproductive functions. Socially acceptable synonyms for these "gutter" words include expressions borrowed from the nursery and the schoolroom, such as *weewee,* *bottom* and *to do number two.* Diarrhea is known by a wide variety of bitterly humorous epithets such as *the runs* and *the trots.* Thomas (7) has assembled a number of popular terms for the ubiquitous and devastating tourist diarrhea, fully half of them containing geographical references. His list includes *Aztec two-step, Casablanca crud, lower Burmas, San Franciscitis, gyppy* (or *Egyptian*) *tummy, Basra belly, Hongkong dog, Montezuma's revenge, Delhi belly, Poona poohs, squitters* and *tourist trots.* Vomiting, too, has its share of slang designations, including *barf, heave, toss, pitch, urp* and *up-chuck.*

Abbreviated forms of medical terms are also popular: *mono* for *mononucleosis, polio* for *poliomyelitis, trich* (or *trick*) for *trichomonal vaginitis* and *flu* for *influenza.* The latter term has a variety of vague and incorrect interpretations, including *gastroenteritis,* any *acute viral syndrome* and indeed any illness whatever characterized by fever and malaise.

Patients occasionally fabricate their own unconventional forms of speech. A diabetic who tells his doctor that he has been "blue for two weeks" may be reporting a bout of depression, but is more likely indicating that his urine has been consistently negative for sugar by the Clinitest tablet method.

Among frankly erroneous lay usages we may waive any consideration of spelling errors. As the patient's spelling of a medical term is much oftener a guess based on something he has heard than a recollection of something he has read, it would scarcely be reasonable to expect a high degree of accuracy in the performance. Moreover, some physicians do not do much better; witness the oft-seen *anuscope, dilitation, innoculate, phalynx, planter.*

Pronunciations that are regionally acceptable (*gooms* for *gums* in the Dakotas and the Ozarks, *fleem* for *phlegm* in Appalachia) may not seem quite appropriate in standard medical English. Errors in pronunciation may be simple phonetic blunders, such as *bronichal, chicken pops,*

7. Thomas C: Gastroenteritis of Travelers in Athletes. American Academy of Orthopaedic Surgeons Symposium on Sports Medicine. St. Louis, CV Mosby, 1969, p 21

clog (for *clot*), *dip'theria, infantigo, prostrate* (for *prostate*), *vomick* and *wound* (for *womb*). But they may also betoken complete misunderstanding of the purport of the word, as in *smilin' mighty Jesus* for *spinal meningitis*. (I have it on excellent authority that this specimen is genuine.) *Gangrene* is often expected to appear green, and *appendix* quite generally regarded as a plural word: "My appendix are out."

Many lay errors represent inaccurate application of anatomic terms. *Stomach,* to perhaps a majority of nonmedical people, means the lower two-thirds of the ventral body surface, while the dorsal body surface is divided by the hips into the *kidneys* and the *base of the spine.* Many seem to take a perverse delight in misapplying the word *base,* speaking of the sacrum as the *base of the spine,* the epigastrium as the *base of the stomach,* the occiput as the *base of the skull* and the cerebellum inside it as the *base of the brain.* The *anus* is generally referred to as the *rectum* and the *vulva* as the *vagina.* The *gallbladder* is frequently confounded with the *urinary bladder,* the spinal *cord* with the spinal *column.*

Schizophrenia is almost universally taken to mean a dual or "split" personality. *Psychosomatic* is frequently truncated to plain *somatic,* which means just the opposite. *Hypertension* (by analogy with *tension*) signifies a chronic anxiety neurosis to many, and *bandage* (by analogy with *Band-Aid*), a dressing or compress. Any laboratory test may be called a *count* ("My uric acid count was high"), any headache is a *migraine,* and any chronic upper respiratory complaint is *sinus* ("I've had sinus for years").

Sulfonamides are often called *sulfur drugs,* and *barbituate* is an extremely common error both in spelling and in pronunciation. Antibiotics are referred to generically as *the mycins,* which more often than not is given an extra syllable, probably by attraction to *niacin,* about which the bread and cereal hucksters are forever babbling on radio and television.

Some inaccuracies probably spring less from ignorance than from exaggeration and a love of the melodramatic. I have seen many patients whose past history included "tearing *all the ligaments* in my knee [or ankle or shoulder]," but fortunately I have never been confronted with such a catastrophe in its acute form.

Patients often express the fear that they have *ptomaine poisoning,* but the medical profession has now abandoned the term, inasmuch as the very existence of ptomaines is in doubt. Though many physicians argue vehemently that the human body contains no such thing as a *solar plexus,* insisting that this must be a mythical structure invented by ringside announcers at boxing matches, the term is simply an outmoded one for the celiac plexus. Some other melodramatic but hideously imprecise terms, which I suspect were concocted originally by the medical profession itself, are *whiplash injury, nervous breakdown* and *low* (or *high*) *pain threshold.*

𝔑ursese

"I wish it was in Jonadge's belly, I do," cried Mrs. *Gamp; appearing to confound the prophet with the whale in this miraculous aspiration.*

Charles Dickens
Martin Chuzzlewit

Between the patient, whose lack of professional training excuses even the most flagrant garbling of medical terms, and the physician, who arrogantly believes that his own usage of these terms should set an inviolable standard, the nurse is trapped in a kind of linguistic limbo. On the one hand she is expected to understand the physician's argot even when it diverges completely from formal terminology, and on the other she is frequently called upon to interpret his cryptic utterances to the patient. Small wonder if her use of technical language sometimes hovers between professional and lay.

For instance, if you ask a nurse whether a razor blade can cause a laceration, or whether tracheal aspiration can relieve congestion, you will probably get an affirmative answer. But a physician would reply that a *laceration,* literally a *tear,* is by definition the result of blunt trauma, whereas a razor blade inflicts an *incised wound.* He would also inform you that *congestion* is a vascular phenomenon, whether nasal, pulmonary, hepatic or elsewhere, and has nothing to do with the presence of excessive secretions. Similarly, the meanings attached by the nurse to *concussion, constipation* and *paranoid* are apt to be closer to the popular definitions of these terms than to the much more specific ones cherished by physicians.

The definition of *crowning,* according to textbooks of obstetrics, is "encirclement of the largest diameter of the fetal head by the vulvar ring." The delivery room nurse, ignoring the metaphorical implications of the word, has changed its meaning to "visibility of the top of the fetal head during a uterine contraction." Indeed, once during my student days I was jolted out of a fitful snooze in the OB lounge by a delivery room nurse's raucous announcement that a patient with a breech presentation was "crowning a foot!"

Nurses also have their own exotic brand of Latin, in which *noc* means *night* (even forming the extraordinary compounds *midnoc* and *tonoc*) and c̄ is used not in the strict pharmaceutical sense of Latin *cum* (of which it is an abbreviation) but in the much broader Germanic sense of *with:* "Area cleansed c̄ soap and water"; "Patient very angry c̄ orderly."

Typistese

phantom word: *A word that came into being through an error of a lexicographer or printer.*
Mario A. Pei and Frank Gaynor
A Dictionary of Linguistics (8)

Even with all its variety and vigor, the language of medicine would be a somewhat dull and sterile idiom were it not for the delicious element of absurdity introduced by the medical records typist. What a boost she can give to the dramatic interest of an operative report by starting it off with the statement, "The patient was prepped and raped in the usual manner"! What zest she can add to an otherwise prosaic and tedious medical history by inserting an expression like "The patient experienced weakness and a pair of seizures in the left lower leg"!

There is a subtle difference between these two examples. The first is probably a typing error, but in the second *a pair of seizures* is a deliberately produced variant rendering of *paresthesias.* It is a matter of no importance whether the dictating physician mumbled or whether the typist simply did not know the word and did her best to come up with a plausible rendering of what she heard. The point is that what she typed was not a mere phonetic transcription, such as *pairuseejuz,* but a legitimate English phrase, which is amusing in this context chiefly because of its incongruity.

Consider another example: "Breath sounds were decreased and residents increased over the entire left chest." Do we not see here the operation of a feeble but genuinely logical effort to make sense out of unintelligible sounds? The trouble is that it is a purely literal logic, such as we might expect of a computer, with horizons no broader than the confines of a single word or phrase. We see that primitive but rigorous "logic" at work in children's mispronunciations based on false

8. Pei MA, Gaynor F: DICTIONARY OF LINGUISTICS. New York, Philosophical Library, 1954

etymology: *ping-wing* for *penguin, lick-stick* for *lipstick, furnastat* for *thermostat.*

It is not my purpose here to disparage the medical records secretary; the vast majority of errors such as I have been describing are undoubtedly traceable to the poor dictating habits of physicians and to the limitations of recording systems. Furthermore, there is no reason to believe that physicians as a class would do a better job of transcribing medical records from dictation, even supposing that they were proficient typists. Indeed, many "variant" spellings originating as errors of medical typists have been picked up and perpetuated by physicians themselves, and a few have practically been canonized by usage: *"shoddy* lymph nodes" and "easy *fatigue ability"* are examples that spring immediately to mind.

7

diseases of the tongue

Introductory Remarks

'Tis hard to say, if greater want of skill
Appear in writing or in judging ill.

Alexander Pope
An Essay on Criticism

Here and there throughout the preceding chapters I have drawn the reader's attention to certain errors that are commonly made in the use of the language of medicine. In this chapter I have brought together a number of such errors for closer scrutiny, fully aware that anyone who sets himself up as a judge of other people's speech and writing habits runs the risk of being condemned himself as a pedant, a purist and a busybody. Instead of the rigid dogmatism that justly merits such judgments, I propose only common sense and practical utility as the criteria for distinguishing "right" from "wrong" in the use of language.

In 1710 Swift (1) wrote, "I would engage to furnish you with a catalogue of English books, published within the compass of seven years past . . . wherein you shall not be able to find ten lines together of common grammar or common sense . . . These two evils, ignorance and want of taste, have produced a third; I mean the continual corruption of the English tongue, which without some timely remedy, will suffer more by the false refinements of twenty years past, than it hath been improved in the foregoing hundred."

John Stuart Mill (2) complained that "Vulgarisms, which creep in nobody knows how, are daily depriving the English language of valu-

1. Swift J: The Tatler, No. 230, September 26, 1710. Presently in print in Scott T (ed): THE PROSE WORKS OF JONATHAN SWIFT, Bohn's Standard Library. London, George Bell & Sons, 1907
2. Mill JS: A SYSTEM OF LOGIC. London, JW Parker, 1843. Current edition: New York, Longmans, Green, 1930

able modes of expressing thought." James Russell Lowell (3) warned against the pernicious example of newspapers: ". . . while the school-master has been busy starching our language and smoothing it flat with the mangle of supposed classical authority, the newspaper reporter has been doing even more harm by stretching and swelling it to suit his occasions." He cites examples of contemporary journalese and utters dire prophecies about their influence on the common speech, asserting that they are "all the more dangerous that their effect, like that of some poisons, is insensibly cumulative, and that they are sure at last of effect among a people whose chief reading is the daily paper."

Many pages might be filled with quotations in the same vein from the writings of editors and authors, critics and scholars. The newest bugbear is television, where, says Hussey (4), "grammatical argot is rife . . . Protection of our youthful ones, those who will speak and write now and in the future, merits attention. Let their parents play a game with the youngsters, taxing [*sic*] them to identify the grammatical aberrations and malapropisms . . . A 20th century crusade for children against the ills of television ill-spoken phrase is needed . . ."

What these well-intentioned but misguided and at times virulent commentators upon language are decrying, one and all, is not illiteracy (the condition in which we are all born) but inelegance in speech and writing. Implicit in the notion of a barbarous or corrupt use of language is the existence of some standard, convention or ideal. The mistake made by many self-appointed custodians of public speech is in confounding the standard of refinement and propriety with the standard of intelligibility. It is not good grammar alone that they want, but good taste (5).

A word or phrase that does not conform to convention may be objectionable because it is imprecise, inaccurate or ambiguous, or on the other hand because it is inelegant, crude or vulgar. But there is not much point in condemning speech that is merely uncouth as "ungrammatical" or "wrong" if it expresses ideas with clarity and precision. I have conversed with thousands of people who habitually used *ain't* to mean *am not, are not, is not, has not* and *have not.* I do not recall a single

3. Lowell JR: BIGLOW PAPERS, second series. Boston, Ticknor & Fields, 1867, Introduction

4. Hussey HH: Television Language: Foster [*sic*] of Illiteracy. JAMA, 228:77, 1974. Copyright 1975, American Medical Association

5. In citing the R. J. Reynolds Tobacco Company as the source of this phrase, I shall refrain from raising the obvious and indeed inevitable question why the public should be forced to choose between grammar and taste instead of having them both.

instance in which I have misunderstood the significance or bearing of the word. Nor is it conceivable that any speaker of English would fail to understand "It don't hurt no more" or "There weren't nothing I could do about it." Logical or not, double negatives are part of the syntactic structure of many languages. We may condemn "If my leg be broke" as rude or uncultured speech, but it is just as intelligible to us as it would have been to Shakespeare's audiences (for it is flawless Elizabethan English). More objectionable by far than these crude but crystal-clear modes of expression are such instances of quasi-scientific gibberish as we shall examine in the following sections.

The common man uses language as a carpenter uses a hammer. It is a tool, indispensable perhaps but after all only a means to an end, and that end is basic workaday communication, not amusement or edification. But though the plain proletarian laboring man, the backbone of civilization, leaves elegance of language to the arty, the academic and the leisured classes, his daily speech has a way of maintaining its intelligibility despite the pernicious example of newspapers, television *and* the inane drivel printed on all six surfaces of breakfast cereal boxes. And it is no wonder. A tool that fails to perform its function is quickly discarded, and words or phrases that do not do the job of communicating are abandoned in favor of others that do.

We can be sure that during the decline of Rome a host of narrow-minded schoolmasters and bookish grammarians spent their time railing at the corruptness and degeneracy of Latin, deploring the loss of inflectional endings in speech and the intrusion of slang words and borrowings from foreign tongues. The writings, and even the names, of these grammarians are lost forever, while the language that was "degenerating" in their time has flowered into modern French, Spanish, Italian, Portuguese and Rumanian. Another crowd of pedantic busybodies sprang up during the Renaissance and took it upon themselves to "correct" the extant manuscripts of the classic writers. Some of them went so far as to amend the colloquialisms and blunders deliberately inserted by the playwrights Plautus and Terence in the speeches of country bumpkins and foreigners.

The fear that obsesses such purists is that the faulty usages of barbarians and uneducated persons will in some way infect the cultured elite and defile their speech as well. It is wildly improbable that persons of sound judgment and clear thought could be spoiled or tainted by contact with speakers of slovenly English. Down through history the most incisive thinkers have generally been the most articulate speakers and writers, and on the other hand it is a matter of common experience that a writer who is incapable of putting together an intelligible paragraph almost never has anything worthwhile to say to his contemporaries, much less to posterity.

Johnson (6) has delineated the role of taste in good writing with characteristic precision and fluency: "Words, being arbitrary, must owe their power to association, and have the influence, and that only, which custom has given them. Language is the dress of thought: and as the noblest mien, or most graceful action, would be degraded and obscured by a garb appropriated to the gross employments of rustics or mechanics; so the most heroic sentiments will lose their efficacy, and the most splendid ideas drop their magnificence, if they are conveyed by words used commonly upon low or trivial occasions, debased by vulgar mouths, and contaminated by inelegant applications . . . Gold may be so concealed in baser metal, that only a chemist can recover it; sense may be so hidden in unrefined and plebeian words, that none but philosophers can distinguish it; and both may be so buried in impurities as not to pay the cost of their extraction."

Having endeavored to make clear the distinction between elegance and mere intelligibility, and without for a moment suggesting that writing which violates the canons of taste and refinement is as good as that which observes them, I relinquish the whole question of style to abler hands. In the succeeding sections of this chapter I propose to concern myself exclusively with modes of speech and writing that are genuinely faulty, that is, that undermine the ability of language to carry out its function, which is the transmission of ideas.

There is no more fundamental or self-evident principle in linguistics than that all language is, in the last analysis, the speech of living persons and is therefore itself a living, changing organism. A dictionary or grammar is a record of the state of the language at a certain time, and quite generally is concerned only with the more fossilized part of the language that constitutes "polite" speech and "formal" writing. Though the dictionary may influence the speaking and writing habits of a few, it can no more prevent the language from changing than a child's photograph can keep him from growing up.

But language is also a convention. When we say *hand* or *hat* or *house* we are using a set of lexical and phonetic conventions inherited from the Anglo-Saxons. When we write these words we employ another set of conventions handed down from the Egyptians and Phoeni-

6. Johnson S: Cowley. In THE LIVES OF THE MOST EMINENT ENGLISH POETS. London, special printing, 1781. Currently available as THE LIVES OF THE ENGLISH POETS, The Everyman Series. Toronto, JM Dent.

cians by way of the Greeks and Romans. When we assert (as we all did in grammar school) that "a relative pronoun is a pronoun that does the work of a conjunction by joining to its antecedent a relative clause of which it is a part," we are acknowledging still another convention. It is, I hope, an axiom requiring no defense that some degree of stability in spelling, pronunciation, punctuation and syntax is essential to intelligibility.

Words are symbols for units of thought, and the construction of a sentence is a problem in applied logic. The only "wrong" solutions to the problem are those that violate intellectual truth; in adjudging certain usages faulty I appeal to no authority or standard other than the judgment of the reader. Despite an almost overpowering temptation to go beyond my brief and inveigh against regrettable popular redefinitions of words like *charisma* and *chauvinism,* to grumble about unidiomatic usages like "He convinced me to operate," and to observe that *boggle* (the latest fad word) is an intransitive verb, I am resolved to confine my observations to modes of expression that are unique to, or at least highly characteristic of, medical speech and writing.

Moreover, I shall refrain from condemning terms and usages that, though repulsive, convey specific ideas clearly, such as the cumbersome adverbs so freely fabricated with *-wise: neurosurgerywise, ST-segmentwise, extracorporeal dialysiswise.* (Like scorpions, these words carry an ugly surprise in their tails.) *Lower-lobed pneumonia* and *left-sided heart failure* are worse than argot—they are vulgar cant, and yet though they affront the hearer's or reader's common sense, they are clearly understood. So are such unlovely inventions as *pallorous, taeniacolic* and *buttocksical,* which, originating as nonce-words, often become established in a physician's working vocabulary and, if he is a teacher, may spread to others around him. Hideous though they are, these words do have plain and simple meanings, and I leave them to those whose ears can tolerate them.

The Wrong Word

Vague and insignificant forms of speech, and abuse of language, have so long passed for mysteries of science: and hard and misapplied words, with little or no meaning, have by prescription, such a right to be taken for deep learning and height of speculation, that it will not be easy to persuade either those who speak or those who hear them,

> *that they are but the covers of ignorance, and hindrance*
> *of true knowledge.*
>
> John Locke
> ***An Essay on Human Understanding***

It is necessary at the outset to distinguish two kinds of speech error: those which are purely verbal, such as mispronunciations or the choice of the wrong one of a pair of similar-sounding words, and those that betoken some deeper confusion of thought. Among purely verbal errors commonly committed by physicians, a few are so deeply entrenched that they generate but little confusion, and indeed scarcely strike the average hearer as errors at all. Among these may be mentioned the expression *flat plate,* which flourishes yet today in the speech of physicians whose parents were not yet born when plates were abandoned for film in medical radiography. *Spasmodic* is often wrongly substituted for *spastic, dose* for *dosage, erectile* for *erect;* and *syndrome = combination of symptoms* is frequently applied to a single symptom or sign.

In many familiar medical expressions, *multiple* is incorrectly used for *many.* English freely forms compounds with *multi–* (*multifocal, multiphasic, multipurpose*) in which the prefix has exactly its original Latin meaning, *many.* But the English adjective *multiple* (from *multi* and *plex =fold*) means not *many* but *manifold,* and its opposite is not *few* but *simple.* The lexical distinction between *many lesions* and *multiple lesions* is essentially the same as that between *four children* and *quadruplets.* In furunculosis there may be *many simple* abscesses; a carbuncle is a *solitary, multiple* abscess. Multifocal PVCs may come from *many,* or *diverse,* or *different,* or *separate,* or *distinct* foci, but they cannot come from *multiple* foci. *Multiple sclerosis* and *multiple myeloma* exemplify correct applications of the word, but such everyday expressions as *multiple syncopal episodes, multiple lumbar punctures* and *multiple psychiatric admissions* are, like the venerable *multiple vitamins,* simply gibberish.

Multiple is a valuable and in fact indispensable word, whose true and exact meaning we are on the verge of losing. It is already too late to salvage such words as *disinterested* and *nauseous.* Though they live on in daily speech, their original denotations now repose on the scrap heap of language, useless alike to the conscientious writer, who dare not use them, and the unsophisticated reader, who has never learned them.

From much wear, adjectives like *marked, substantial, considerable* and *moderate* have come to be almost meaningless. They are rendered even more nearly so by constructions like "On admission the patient displayed moderate to marked dyspnea." It is impossible to justify, much less interpret, the adverbs in such common expressions as *predominantly unchanged* and *essentially unremarkable.*

Negative expressions in particular tend to lose their force and even their meaning after much repetition and misapplication. A sound rule for the writing of accurate as well as readable clinical records is to avoid as completely as possible the word *normal.* "The skin is normal" might be substituted for either of the following descriptions, but with a regrettable sacrifice of precision and detail: "The skin is deeply tanned on surfaces not covered by street clothes, warm to the touch, and of good turgor"; "The skin is pale, cool and slightly moist, and there are several small senile keratoses on the upper back."

Avoidance of this word will also help the physician steer clear of such absurdities as "Homans' sign is normal" and "The Queckenstedt test is normal." A sign is either *present* or *absent,* and the outcome of a diagnostic maneuver is either *positive* or *negative,* but neither can properly be reported as *normal.*

An undue reliance on negative expressions can rob a written record of much of its validity. Carefully consider the following excerpt from a physical examination report: "Examination of the heart disclosed no arrhythmia; no heave, shock, or thrill; no murmurs or abnormal heart sounds; no evidence of cardiomegaly; no pericardial friction rub." Is there anything in these remarks to indicate whether the heart was actually beating at the time of the examination? Negatives to be particularly eschewed are *noncontributory* and *unremarkable.* All too often, the first means "I didn't ask" and the second, "I didn't look."

By contrast with the insipidity and vacuousness of worn-out words and negative expressions, the language of medicine includes a few adjectives that go to the opposite extreme. Long-established usage has brought into acceptance a remarkable variety of melodramatic expressions like *florid cirrhosis* and *frank pus.* It is an everyday experience to hear (or read) such remarks as "Intravenous gentamycin brought about a dramatic lowering of fever." There is nothing dramatic about a drug's performing its intended function, and in this instance neither the rate nor the degree of defervescence can have been so far beyond the physician's expectations as to justify the use of the word. *Fulminant renal failure* is also something of an exaggeration, since *fulminant* means *with the speed of lightning. Massive* should probably be dropped from the physician's professional vocabulary; not only is there a certain incongruity in the notion of *massive fluid replacement,* but it seems ridiculous to describe as *massive* a dose measured in milligrams or a thrombus measured in millimeters.

The sense of *increased* and *decreased* when applied to physical findings is often hard to pin down. In "Auscultation revealed decreased breath sounds," one would suppose that the auscultator is making a comparison with what he heard during a previous examination of the same patient; yet this is clearly not the case in "Auscultation of the newborn immediately after delivery revealed decreased breath sounds over the entire left chest." The fact is that *increased, decreased, reduced* and *diminished* generally imply a comparison with some abstract standard of normalcy, not with a previous state of the patient being examined.

Certain other common usages, though they may escape the accusation of absolute unintelligibility, are nonetheless objectionable because they cast more shadow than light. In the expression *delusional-like ideation,* the effort to produce an adjective from a noun has been a little overdone, for either *delusion-like* or *delusional* would suffice, though of course there is a shade of difference between the two. Similarly, either *sleep-like state* or *hypnoid state* would be preferable to *hypnoid-like state.*

The custom of reporting the dimensions of a tumor or other mass by comparing it to a familiar article such as a hen's egg or a cherrystone is occasionally the object of mild reproof from medical educators and medical editors. One objection to this practice is that many such articles (lemons, potatoes) vary greatly in size; another is that some of them (pomegranate seeds, plover's eggs) may not be equally familiar to all.

The classicist makes a sour face when he hears someone speak of a *bottomless abyss* because he knows that the idea *bottomless* is inherent in the word *abyss.* Likewise, he objects to *a mural on the wall* because *on the wall* is just exactly what *mural* means. But though he strains at these tautologies, he is likely to swallow others of equal redundancy, like *private secretary* and *yellow jaundice.* Our acceptance or rejection of redundant expressions depends upon how literally we interpret the words we use, and also upon the variant meanings that convention has assigned to them. It is possible that *edematous swelling* may occasionally be justified (as distinguished from swelling due to hemorrhage, for example), but *traumatic injury, cervical collar, cut section* and *walled-off abscess* are all indefensible, since the adjective in each case merely repeats, or rather anticipates, the idea inherent in the noun. *PZI insulin* is likewise redundant, since *PZI* stands for *protamine zinc insulin.*

Both plain English and medical terminology contain many nouns ending in *–escence.* Most of them have corresponding adjectives in *–escent* and some have verbs, produced by back-formation, in *–esce.* Some of these words are descended directly from Latin verbs of the class known as inceptives or inchoatives, and the rest have been formed in modern times on the same pattern. The Latin verb-ending *–escere* signalizes a word meaning *becoming* or *beginning to be: adolescere*=*to* *become adult; senescere=to grow old.* Though a few modern words like *fluorescence* and *phosphorescence* are exceptions to the rule, *–escence* words in general should be regarded as meaning *becoming* or denoting a *change of state.* Hence *coalescence* means *a going together,* but does not properly indicate the condition of things already completely joined or intermingled. *To become defervescent, to grow tumescent* and *to remain quiescent* are solecisms.

Losing sight of the original purport of words can also result in self-contradictory expressions like this one, which appears in a distinguished medical manual: "The more indolent forms of pericarditis (tuberculous, uremic) may be free of pain." By definition, anything that is *indolent* in the medical sense is altogether *free of pain.* Probably there can be little objection nowadays to *axillary buboes,* though *bubo* comes from the Greek word for *groin.* Similarly, *retrograde ejaculation* is sufficiently intelligible even though the noun specifically means *a casting out.* Few if any medical journals have ever been published *daily,* though that is the literal meaning of *journal. Patient (=one who is suffering)* is not a very apposite designation for a visitor to a well-child clinic (except when immunizations are due).

A favorite target of the language purist is the dangling modifier, as exemplified in "Dissecting laterally, the thyroid was separated from its capsule." We shall see more of this kind of construction later, but here we shall take a look at a particular species of dangling modifier, which might be designated the half-baked connective.

From the standpoint of language evolution, connectives (prepositions and conjunctions) can be divided into three general categories. Primitive connectives express fundamental relationships and are simple in form: *to, of, and, but.* Derived connectives express more complex relationships and often retain the form of some other part of speech, usually an adjective or participle, from which they have evolved: *during, provided, according to.*

A great many expressions in common speech are in a third class, a sort of limbo between erroneous usage and full acceptance as derived connectives. It is not my purpose to reactivate the battles over the use of *like* and *due to* as conjunctions. But even with the most liberal and indulgent attitude toward these apprentice connectives, we cannot ignore the fact that they sometimes fall down on the job. The substitution of adjectives like *prior* and *subsequent,* or participles like *following* or *based on,* for full-fledged prepositions and conjunctions may be justified in speech, because the intonation given to the words makes their function more obvious than if they were being read. But the habitual use of these words in speech leads inevitably to shoddy habits of writing, and we encounter absurdities in print like "A twenty-seven-year-old white male was seen in the outpatient department following a prize fight." Worse, we find occasional sentences in which no amount of rereading and reflection enables us to decide whether an adjective is to be taken at face value or has been pressed into service as a connective: "Aspirin is well known to inhibit secondary platelet aggregation due to interference with release of intrinsic adenosine diphosphate." To object that any confusion here could have been obviated by putting a comma after *aggregation* not only is inaccurate but goes no further toward justifying this kind of construction than the observation that if the reader knew his biochemistry he would understand the passage readily enough.

Equally ambiguous is this statement in the manufacturer's literature about an anabolic steroid: "The only absolute contraindication is carcinoma of the prostate due to the androgenic activity of [the drug]." Here again, setting off the floating *due to* phrase with a comma would have done little to resolve the confusion.

A relative upstart among half-baked connectives is the dangling participle *based on:* "The drug is not subject to narcotic controls, based on the results of findings in direct addiction tests." This pattern of usage is heard with increasing frequency, and has lately been introduced into the formula "Based on a review of this drug by the National Academy of Sciences—National Research Council and/or other information, FDA has classified the indications as follows," which keeps recurring, like a sort of comic chorus, throughout the two-thousand-and-odd pages of the *Physicians' Desk Reference.*

Latin and Greek

Besides, 'tis known he could speak Greek
As naturally as pigs squeak:
That Latin was no more difficile
Than to a blackbird 'tis to whistle.
Being rich in both, he never scanted
His bounty unto such as wanted
But much of either would afford
To many that had not one word.

Samuel Butler
Hudibras

Medical terms derived from the classic languages can be divided into two main groups. The first comprises those that are either Anglicized forms of Latin or Greek words, like *clavicle* and *rickets,* or English words built from Latin or Greek stems, like *retrosternal* and *cystoscope.* These words are strictly English in form and are handled as such by speakers and writers of English.

The other group includes those words and expressions that preserve the original form of the Latin or (usually Latinized) Greek word: *serosa, rhonchus, femur, syncope, asterixis, flexor digitorum profundus* and *pulsus rarus, parvus et tardus.* Though many of the expressions in this class have been thoroughly naturalized, so that we treat them just as though they were English words, others preserve a distinctly foreign character. We can, for instance, speak of *adductors* or *fistulas,* but it is hard to imagine that any professional person, even one totally ignorant of Latin, would dare to say *corpus cavernosums.*

This example pinpoints both of the challenges that English-speaking physicians must meet in using terms that preserve their Latin or Greek form: the correct handling of phrases and the proper formation of plurals(7). Because English has few inflections, persons whose mother tongue is English are likely to be impatient with the grammatical rules of inflected languages, and inept at learning and applying them. A common error is the ungrammatical combination of a noun and an adjective; in a single day I ran across *pyoderma gangrenosa, sinus tarsus, Treponema pallida* and *vasa vasora,* all in print and all wrong.

The linguistically naive, misled by such everyday expressions as *vena cava, situs inversus,* and *stratum corneum,* are apt to conclude that matching nouns to adjectives in Latin is merely a matter of rhyming. Unfortunately it is not so simple as that. An adjective must "agree" with its noun in gender (and number and case), but the gender of any given inflectional ending is not absolutely fixed. For example, though most Latin nouns ending in *–us* are masculine, *corpus* and *pectus* are neuter, while *manus* and, of course, *Venus* are feminine. The adjectives *planus* and *sclerosus* are masculine, but *minus* and *majus* are neuter. Again, though most Latin nouns ending in *–a* are feminine, some that have been borrowed from Greek are neuter *(enema, soma, stoma)* and such words as *strata* and *milia* are plural forms of neuter nouns ending in *–um.*

Pyoderma and *Treponema,* both Greek-derived neuter nouns, re-

7. It is not my purpose in these pages to offer a crash course in medical Latin. For detailed information on Latin accidence, the reader is referred to the excellent set of tables in the introductory pages of STEDMAN'S MEDICAL DICTIONARY.

quire the neuter adjectives *gangrenosum* and *pallidum*. In *sinus tarsi =
cavity of the ankle* the second word is not an adjective but another noun;
vasa vasorum = vessels of the vessels also consists of two nouns, or rather
of one noun in two different forms. The adjectives *varus* and *valgus*
change their terminations to agree in gender with the noun modified
(*pes varus, genu varum, coxa vara*), so that it is not strictly correct to speak
of "varus deformity of the knee."

It is considered good *English* usage to say and write *fetuses;* the
incorrect Latin plural *feti* only betrays the ignorance of the speaker. But
there are objections to forming the plurals of all "foreign" words by
adding *–s* or *–es*. This practice would be a sore disappointment to the
pedants who glory in such plurals as *encephalitides* and *enemata*. Moreover, no one is likely to take kindly to expressions like *analysises of renal
calculuses* or *neurosises and psychosises*. If, however, the correct plurals are
to be used, physicians need to know enough Latin and Greek to avoid
such blunders as *decubiti* and *pruritides*.

Latin nouns ending in *–a* quite consistently form their plurals in
–ae: herniae, scapulae. Many Greek nouns ending in *–a* have joined this
class in becoming Latinized: *pleurae, tracheae*. But when the final *–a* of
a Greek noun is preceded by *m*, the word is usually a third declension
neuter, which forms its plural in *–ata (stomata, condylomata)*.

Many Greek and nearly all Latin nouns ending in *–is* form their
plurals by changing *–is* to *–es*, (*paralyses, pelves*) but in a few Greek
words the stem undergoes a more elaborate change: *epididymides, arthri-
tides*.

A Latin noun ending in *–us* may belong to the second, the third
or the fourth declension, each of which forms its plurals in a different
way. Nouns of the second declension, such as *villus* and *limbus,* form
the plural in *–i: villi, limbi*. Greek nouns ending in *–os* usually join this
group: *bronchus, borborygmus, canthus*. A few Greek compounds ending
in *–pous = foot* have joined it also, and though we have Anglicized
polypus by cutting off the Latin termination, we still sometimes hear the
plural *polypi,* which is perfectly correct if a little archaic. (*Octopi,* however, is a variant that the dictionaries will not tolerate in place of the
classic *octopodes,* though most of them permit *octopuses*.)

Latin nouns of the third declension that end in *–us* form their
plurals by changing *s* to *r* (often changing the preceding vowel as well)
and generally ending in *–a: corpus, corpora; crus, crura; pectus, pectora; pus,
pura*.

A relatively large class of Latin nouns in *–us* belong to the fourth
declension. Many of these are formed directly from verbs and are

known in Latin grammar as supines: *decubitus, ductus, fetus, fremitus, ictus, meatus, pruritus, risus, tinnitus, vomitus.* The plurals of nouns in this group are spelled exactly like the singulars. The Romans made a distinction between the two forms in speech, but exactly how they pronounced either form is and always will be a puzzle for the experts to worry about. A more practical question is how we can retain the correct spelling and avoid misunderstanding.

The French form plurals by adding an *s* which is seldom pronounced, but in the spoken language the preceding article indicates whether the noun is singular or plural. We have no such arrangement, but we manage pretty well with words like *series, species* and *sheep,* whose singular and plural forms are identical. Probably the best solution is to follow the practice of forming the plural of a fourth declension Latin noun by adding *–es,* as in *fetuses.* Fortunately, words like *pruritus* and *tinnitus* are not often used in the plural.

Some Latin terms appear to be singular though they are actually plural *(excreta, genitalia, milia, strata),* while others that are singular look like plurals because they end in *s (ascites, biceps, herpes, scabies).* Though grammatically singular, *forceps* has so long been taken for a plural form ("a pair of forceps," "these forceps are contaminated") that it may as well be one; it is futile to argue against the example of true plurals like *scissors, pliers, tweezers* and the like.

A frequent source of error is faulty back-formation of a singular from a word that is usually used in the plural. Most physicians are above saying *varice* for *varix* or *nare* for *naris* (though they may take the easy way out by substituting *varicosity* and *nostril* for the Latin singulars). But certain parallel mistakes are almost universal. The nonexistent words *comedone* and *fomite* can be found in any number of authoritative texts and reference works. The correct singular of *fomites* (three syllables) is *fomes,* just as the correct singulars of *comedones, meninges* and *feces* are *comedo, meninx* and *fex.*

Rhagades is a plural for which no singular form exists, and *sordes* can be either singular or plural. *Sputa* is a formally correct plural of *sputum,* but in the sentence "Sputa grew pure cultures of *Serratia marcescens,*" it serves merely as a careless and slightly silly abbreviation for *specimens of sputum.*

It is often argued that the rules of a dead language should exercise no influence over English usage. The modern savant insists upon his right to say "This data is inadequate" and "That media is contaminated" with utter disregard for the fact that *data* and *media* are plural. But surely it is irrational and absurd to cling to a system of nomenclature as tenaciously as modern medicine clings to its quite extensive hoard of Latin, and yet refuse to observe the fundamental principles governing its use.

Worse than the speaker or writer who knows nothing about the classic languages is the one who mistakenly believes he knows everything about them. He can be recognized easily by his habit of saying *cicatrix, facies* and *singultus* instead of *scar, face* and *hiccups,* and by the unction with which he mouths such modern jargon words as *cor bovinum, sensorium* and *status anginosus,* which would have baffled not only Celsus but Harvey and Lister as well. He and others of his kind are responsible for the fabrication of pseudo-Latin words like *precordium* (derived by back-formation from *precordial* and now substituted for classic *praecordia*) and *hilus* (a superfluous variant of *hilum*). He will discourse learnedly on *iris,* the Latin word for *ring,* though *iris* is Greek for *rainbow.* He will tell you that *Pyrex* glass is named after the Greek word for *fire,* though it is really so styled because it was developed as a material for making pie pans.

Sometimes, when he has imbibed a little too freely the heady wine of fragmentary knowledge, the amateur classicist grows so hardy and arrogant as to fashion "Latin" expressions anew. The fruits of his genius are often howlers worthy of a stage farce; *fetor garlicosis, pulsus paradoxus pulmonale* and *acne detergicans* (8) are fit not merely to break Priscian's head but to pulverize every bone in his body.

Pronunciation

> *The pronunciation is the actual living form or forms of a word, that is, the word itself,* of which the current spelling is only a symbolization—generally, indeed, only the traditionally-preserved symbolization of an earlier form, sometimes imperfect to begin with, still oftener corrupted in its passage to our time.
>
> *A New English Dictionary (Oxford),*
> *Introduction*

8. Like nearly all the specimens of aberrant usage in this book, these are actual examples taken from the recent medical literature. To cite references for all of these blunders and inadvertencies would be to malign and offend a good many writers and editors of undoubted merit, and at the risk of being accused of fabricating them all to suit my purposes, I shall not identify the sources of my specimens.

I do not propose to venture very far into this subject, though I might fill a page or two with bitter denunciations of those barbarians who say *abscesseez, aceedic, dysect* and *larnyx.* The English language community is so vast and variegated that one must be circumspect indeed in laying down rules for pronunciation. One unfortunate trait of American speech, which is perhaps only an extension of a characteristic to be found in the Queen's English as well, is its tolerance of what may be called the neutral vowel sound, represented by the *a* in *oral,* the *e* in *liver,* the *i* in *urine,* the *o* in *tumor* and the *u* in *fetus. Appellation* is pronounced exactly like *Appalachian, principal* like *principle, perineal* like *peroneal, aural* like *oral. Austin* rhymes with *Boston* and *hapten* with *captain.*

A special instance of this homophony involves nouns ending in *–us* and their derivative adjectives in *–ous.* Common errors in spelling arising from confusion of the two forms include *mucus membrane, a plug of mucous, villus adenoma* and *ruptured viscous.* In the case of *callus* an interesting development has occurred. The noun is quite generally misspelled *callous* (9), and from this "stem" a new adjective, *calloused,* has been manufactured to fill the place that *callous* itself should occupy. Not only is *calloused* (used ordinarily only in the figurative sense of *hard-hearted*) a vulgarism, but it happens to sound exactly like *callused,* a legitimate word meaning *having a callus.* The confusion has driven some speakers and writers to discard the original word altogether and employ instead the cumbersome derivative *callosity.*

As a rule we apply English principles of pronunciation even to words taken bodily from foreign languages: *hematoma, rabies, stab cell* and *alkali* are all pronounced as though they were Anglo-Saxon words. Though the British observe rather strictly the so-called "reformed" pronunciation of Latin and Greek terms (which assigns to the vowels in these languages sounds that it is more than probable the Romans and Greeks of antiquity never gave them), contemporary American medical parlance follows no discernible pattern. Classic rules for the placement of accent are generally ignored. For example, though in *saliva, pruritus* and *diarrhea* the stress is placed where it belongs, on the second-last syllable, it has been wrongly shifted forward in the accepted modern pronunciations of *gingiva, tinnitus* and *trachea.* A double example of the reverse "error" is seen in the popular pronunciation *anGIna pecTORis.*

Although borrowings from most modern foreign languages are treated as though they were native English words, French terms consti-

9. Even Dr. Scholl sells *callous* (not *callus*) pads.

tute a curious exception to the rule. Of course, *tache cérébrale* and *tic douloureux* are so obviously foreign that it is no wonder if we try to preserve something of their original intonation. But such words as *lavage* and *massage*, despite the example of *ravage* and *message*, are customarily given a French sound also.

In many instances the approach to authentic French pronunciation is not very close. The French say *bruit* and *chancre* as words of one syllable. *Petty mal* is a corrupt pronunciation, reminiscent of Law French terms like *petty larceny* and *petty jury.* Though the last letter or two of a French word are often silent, *malaise* and *buret* (which is a cropped form of *burette*) correctly end with *s (z)* and *t* sounds respectively. On the other hand, *facet,* though originally French, was long ago naturalized as an English word, and should be pronounced FASSet; the oft-heard faSET is neither English nor French.

Besides displaying a strong tendency to preserve something like the correct pronunciation in borrowings from French, physicians seem to delight in forcing this pronunciation on words that are not French at all. For example, we often hear the Latin adjectives *mitrale, ovale* and *pulmonale* pronounced to rhyme with *morale* and *chorale,* apparently on the supposition that like the latter terms they have been borrowed from French. *Annulare, inguinale* and *multiforme* are also Latin, and the final *e*'s are therefore pronounced. Though *scalpel* and *vaccine* are commonly accented on the second syllable as though they were French, both came directly from Latin.

Raphe, too, which is Greek, should be accented on the first syllable rather than the second. *Macrophage* and *bacteriophage* are not infrequently made to rhyme with *lavage,* though the stem –*phage* is also Greek. *Chalazion* may look French but is pure Greek *(chalaza = pimple),* and the *ch* should be given a *k* sound.

Words beginning with *cent–* seem particularly susceptible to this obsessive Gallicization. *Centigrade, centimeter* and *centrifuge* are all English words coined directly from the classic languages; there is nothing French about them, though to be sure the French have essentially the same words in their language. Even if these were borrowings from French, pronouncing their first syllables to rhyme with *John* would be a pathetically feeble effort in the direction of giving them an authentic French sound. Some *précieux ridicules* even go so far as to say *eosahnophil* and *sahntillation counter.*

When the typical slapdash Frenchifier encounters a real French expression he often botches the pronunciation completely. To a Frenchman, the letter *y* is a "Greek *i*" *(i grec),* so that the usual American pronunciation of *Roux en-Y* [*anastomosis*] as *roo-awn-wye* is a bit wide of the mark.

𝕸𝖚𝖉𝖉𝖞 𝖂𝖆𝖙𝖊𝖗𝖘

> *Only those whose thoughts are accurate and well-disciplined attain to the highest degree of linguistic precision.*
>
> Otto Jespersen
> *Growth and Structure of the English Language* (10)

The faults of speech that we have considered hitherto are such as even a physician of genius and perspicuity may occasionally fall into, for they are, after all, purely verbal errors arising from some lapse or flaw in the reproduction of a conventional symbol. It is not always possible to distinguish between errors due merely to slovenly habits of speech and those that indicate slovenly habits of thought.

The workaday speech of physicians and nonphysicians alike is apt to become so cluttered with formulas and clichés as to enfeeble every assertion to the point of insipidity. If a screwdriver is used as a chisel, a scraper, a nail-puller, a pry-bar and a can opener, it will soon be unable to fulfill the purpose for which it was made. So the lexical value and specificity of a word are diluted and weakened in proportion to the number and variety of connotations in which it is forced to serve.

Almost any word or phrase, if repeated often enough, can become a formula to which the mind attaches little if any of its literal meaning. The formula then becomes the master, and betrays the speaker into one absurdity after another. Language has completely taken leave of thought in sentences like "The urine was grossly bloody and showed four-plus occult blood" or "Palpation of the prostate revealed the prostate to be surgically absent," and it is hard to put much faith in the diagnostic acumen, or even the sanity, of a physician who is capable of expressing himself in these ways.

But if these examples represent, after all, merely extreme instances of the tyranny of words and the carelessness of tired or hurried people, there are other kinds of language abuse that cannot so readily be excused. Astonishing as it may seem, there are professional people who

10. Jespersen O: GROWTH AND STRUCTURE OF THE ENGLISH LANGUAGE, 9th ed. Riverside, NJ, The Free Press, MacMillan, 1968

can perceive absolutely no difference between "An absent enzyme resulted in decreased efficiency" and "The absence of an enzyme resulted in a decrease of efficiency." These are the same people who diagnose "impending liver failure," who aver that "involvement of the eye by mycosis fungoides is usually quite rare," and who throw around frankly self-contradictory phrases like "hazardous safety conditions."

One of the commonest of these forms of double-talk is that which results when an intangible quality is concretized by being absorbed into something tangible, as when the patient says, "My sore throat went away and my upset stomach is gone." Study these sentences carefully: "Tetany was due to decreased serum calcium." "Auscultation of the left chest revealed absent breath sounds." Both statements are clearly intelligible to the medical man, who is accustomed to such conventions, and yet there is a certain disquieting fuzziness about them. Tetany cannot be due to calcium, no matter by what adjectives we choose to qualify the latter word. Auscultation may reveal the absence of something, but can hardly reveal that which is absent. The speakers of these sentences have allowed their mental gears to slip, with the result that the composite concepts *decreased-serum-calcium* and *absent-breath-sounds* have been transferred bodily into speech, where they serve formal roles that violate not only the rules of syntax but also common sense.

Similar instances of concretization occur in "The patient suffered a *fractured femur*" and "Infection no doubt played a part in the *poor control* of his diabetes." Still another example is seen in "An alert and oriented patient may or may not indicate that treatment was successful," where the speaker, in order to avoid the slightly cumbersome "alertness and orientation of the patient," has run headlong into nonsense.

The concept of rate, being a derived and intangible one, is sometimes concretized by being absorbed into that of time, which is a little less abstract. When this occurs, the result is often a complete change of meaning. "Swallowed barium appeared in the colon in twenty-five minutes, indicating an increased transit time": what the radiologist means is an increased *rate* of transit, with resultant shortening of transit time. "Cervical cytology should be repeated at least yearly": the pathologist does not mean that a year is the least recommended interval, but that a rate of one examination a year is the least recommended frequency.

Analogous errors creep into speech and writing about quantitative determinations in which a time factor is used to measure a concentration. Thus, the expression *decreased prothrombin time* is often incorrectly substituted for *decreased prothrombin activity,* which is reflected in a prolongation of the prothrombin time. These aberrations are reminiscent of Madison Avenue gibberish ("twice as few calories," "four times as low in saturated fats"), to whose example they perhaps owe their origin.

𝔙𝔢𝔯𝔟𝔬𝔰𝔦𝔱𝔶

Words are like leaves; and where they most abound,
Much fruit of sense beneath is rarely found.

Alexander Pope
An Essay on Criticism

As we have been concerned until now chiefly with blunders committed in speech, and as I intend to take up briefly, in the next section, the subject of medical writing, this seems a fitting place to discuss a disorder of language that has its roots in faulty speech habits but crops up to taint and disfigure much written material as well.

Every physician has heard an adolescent patient say things of this sort: "Like I like fell on it and it like hurts if I like press on it." This is of course simply a bad speech habit picked up from peers, and yet it is generally evident that it has a way of justifying and even exacerbating vagueness of thought. One may well use a qualifying expression such as *sort of* or *kind of* or *like* when he is reluctant to make an absolute assertion, but when the word *like* appears three or four times in every sentence that a person speaks, it is plain that he either suffers from a kind of universal uncertainty or is afflicted with a disorder of the process by which thought is transmuted into speech.

To take a more extreme example, consider the species of cerebral stuttering that one hears on the execrable "open microphone" or "talk" shows of radio and television: "I mean, you know, I mean, I don't know, I think—I don't think you can, you know, really say it's —I mean, OK, sure, if you want to call it that, but to say, you know what I mean . . ." Whereas the child who habitually punctuates his sentences with *like* generally manages to fit a certain amount of intelligible language in among the superfluous words, this "interviewee" has produced an elaborate tissue of verbiage that means absolutely nothing.

Words and phrases of nebulous significance and equivocal bearing are unfortunately popular in medical speech and writing, where they serve a variety of roles. In the last chapter we mentioned jargon words like *factor, aspect* and *parameter,* which can mean practically anything.

The speaker who uses vague and noncommittal terms like these seems to consider himself absolved from thinking clearly or nailing down definitions and distinctions either in his mind or in his utterances.

In the last section of the present chapter we saw instances of words and phrases that have been battered by overuse into hollow, worthless clichés. These expressions are wonderfully convenient devices for the writer who wants to swell out a phrase into a sentence or a sentence into a paragraph but cannot be troubled to give the reader a full tally of meaning. What is the exact significance and purpose of the italicized words in the expressions "disease *entity*," "treatment *modality*," "*clinical* disorder," "*clinical entity*"? In the first three examples what, if anything, is lost by expunging the non-word? What, if anything, does the last expression mean?

Clinical is one of the most hackneyed and useless terms in the entire language of medicine. It is impossible to formulate an exact definition that will accurately represent its meaning in all of the following expressions: *clinical judgment, clinical improvement, clinical thermometer, clinical pathology, clinical death, clinical trial, subclinical infection.*

Why does a writer refer to "health care of the individual patient?" *Individual* here contributes nothing; its role as a qualifier of *patient* is purely illusory, for the writer inserted it only because he felt the need to justify the phrase *of the patient,* which is itself superfluous. Who else could be the object of health care? "Heart block and existing congestive failure are major contraindications to the use of propranolol." The notion of existence is inherent in the meaning of every noun. Surely it is pointless to qualify congestive failure as *existing,* for if it did not exist it could not be a contraindication to anything, and indeed would not even bear mentioning.

Superfluous and noncommittal words and phrases like these are so many parasitic excrescences, choking the life and sapping the vigor of plain, honest English. No less objectionable is the pompous practice of using long or arcane words where shorter and plainer ones would be more appropriate. An article written in this bloated and ungainly style can usually be recognized from its very first sentence, which warns the experienced reader against proceeding further. Though this species of prolixity may be merely a bad habit, in many instances the technique seems to be deliberately chosen to lend an air of scholarship and erudition to pedestrian writing.

A second motive may be a mania for synonyms, or more accurately a horror of repeating a word. Almost the highest praise that a French or Spanish literary critic can bestow upon the prose style of one of his countrymen is to call it simple, lucid and precise. If these languages lack the flexibility and variety of English, they are also free of many of the snares and pitfalls that English can lay for the unwary and unpracticed writer. Because they are not so rich as English in synonyms and acceptable variant forms, in these languages the repetition of a word several times in a single paragraph is not viewed as a fault of style. In English, on the other hand, such repetition is a cardinal sin, and in struggling to avoid it many writers of small capacity commit the even worse blunder of trotting out a whole string of synonyms borrowed straight from Roget's THESAURUS or Hartrampf's VOCABULARIES. Though some of these variations may be in keeping with good formal usage, others will be archaic, colloquial, stilted or jocular. Journalists, particularly sports writers, are notoriously prone not only to fall into this practice, but to cling to it and cultivate it as if it were a talent instead of a fault. Many medical writers evidently labor under the same delusion.

𝔐𝔢𝔡𝔦𝔠𝔞𝔩 𝔚𝔯𝔦𝔱𝔦𝔫𝔤

> *Oh, for one man who should write healthy, hearty,*
> *straightforward English!*
>
> Hilaire Belloc
> *The Path to Rome (11)*

The canons of good writing are necessarily different and more strict than those governing speech. The speaker has at his command a whole battery of devices, including gestures and facial expressions, intonation, emphasis and phrasing, with which to qualify the bare meaning of his words. Moreover, in most instances the speaker can observe at once whether his meaning is clear to his auditors, and if it is not he can restate his ideas until he is understood.

By contrast, the writer, who must make do with a few punctuation marks to break up the mass of his discourse into intelligible morsels, is held to a much narrower range of variations in sentence structure and word order. As his work may and perhaps ought to survive him by many decades, and pass far beyond the bounds of his own speech community, he should spare no pains to outfit his ideas in the most durable material available to him: clear and precise English. Let skeptics

11. Belloc H: THE PATH TO ROME. New York, Image, 1956

ransack the libraries; they will discover that nearly every work that has endured for more than a generation is conspicuous for the purity and propriety of its language.

Faults of medical writing, when they do not consist simply of a reproduction of speech faults such as we have discussed in the foregoing sections, can nearly all be reduced to either obscurity or inelegance. I have already stated elsewhere that I propose to limit myself to a consideration of how vague and muddled language can be made plain, without inquiring how plain language can be made fancy. Though a piece of writing that is frankly ugly can fail to perform its function if it repels the reader before he has penetrated far enough into it to digest its meaning, obscurity in writing is a far more serious fault than mere clumsiness.

Perhaps ambiguity would be a better word than obscurity in this context. Generally the reader of a medical article or textbook has some knowledge of the subject matter already, and he has the advantage over the reader of fiction or poetry that he can usually take it for granted that the writer means *something.* His plight, then, is more likely to be an uncertainty which of two or more possible interpretations to follow than a complete lack of understanding.

Ambiguity in writing may arise from a variety of causes. Naturally, it may be the consequence of simple ineptitude or carelessness, and yet many skilled and painstaking writers have produced occasional passages of double-talk. Even great Osler nods, as when he suggests that in cases of pyelonephritis suspected of being tuberculous, "intraperitoneal injections of guinea pigs should also be made." (12) As in most of the specimens of equivocal writing that we are about to examine, the confusion here is only momentary.

Much of the obscurity that one finds in technical writing can be attributed to genuine errors of grammar and syntax. Consider the following examples:

"Mononucleosis is a disease caused by a virus which occurs almost exclusively in teenagers and young adults."

"Erythrocytes which contain iron pigment can also yield a positive reaction."

"Gout is a condition from which no one should suffer because of advances in specific biochemical therapy."

These are "textbook" examples of sentences from which commas have been wrongly omitted. Though one or two of them display other

12. Osler W: THE PRINCIPLES AND PRACTICE OF MEDICINE, 7th ed. New York, D. Appleton & Co., 1909, p 706

stylistic faults as well, they could all be made more accurate and intelligible by the appropriate addition of commas. Generally the symbol of a pause, the comma by convention also sets off nonrestrictive phrases and clauses like *which contain iron pigment* in the second sentence above. If this sentence were taken at face value, the inference would be that some erythrocytes do not contain iron pigment. (13)

The usage exemplified in these sentences is objectionable not because it violates a rule that appears in all grammar books, but because it violates truth and reason. By and large, rules of grammar, syntax and punctuation are valid only insofar as they protect the integrity of thought and prevent confusion and inaccuracy of expression. In sharp contrast to the writers quoted at the beginning of this chapter, Barzun (14) sounds a note of sanity and practicality: ". . . The whole force of one's objection to another's writing must first be directed at the failure to represent the truth . . . The whole effort of an editor must be to convince the writer that slipshod expression is as grave an error as wrong figures, wrong names, wrong middle initials."

Another species of syntactic flaw that leads to ambiguity is what may be termed the midsentence thought shift. Every sentence may be conceived as having a certain axis or polarity, which is determined by the main subject and predicate, as in

The patient——————complained.

Other words and phrases added to this skeleton or framework must take their orientation from the principal axis. That, however, is just what they do not do in the following elaboration: "Advancing the probe under fluoroscopic control to the opposite margin of the cavity, the patient suddenly complained of a severe, stabbing pain." The participial phrase that begins the sentence creates an altogether false setting for the main clause, which contains nothing that the participle can logically qualify, limit or describe. For one brief moment before comprehension dawns we are struck by the grimly ludicrous impression that it is the patient himself who is advancing the probe.

The dangling participle is a peculiarly English fault, and it has recurred down through the centuries to mar and muddle the writing

13. Though in English the comma is invariably the sign of a nonrestricting phrase or clause (as in "My nose, which sometimes bleeds") this is only a convention. In German all relative clauses, restricting or not, are set off by commas, whereas in French the comma is often omitted even with nonrestricting clauses.

14. Barzun J: So Long As Doctors Have to Think. Bull NYAM 47:229, 1971. Professor Barzun has done as much as any man living to foster, by both precept and example, healthy habits of speech and writing.

of some of the greatest lights of English literature. But other things than participles may dangle and require shifts of thought in midsentence. Consider this passage from Edward Gibbon's AUTOBIOGRAPHY: "Instead of guiding the studies, and watching over the behavior of his disciple, I was never summoned to attend even the ceremony of a lecture; and, excepting one voluntary visit to his rooms, during the eight months of his titular office the tutor and pupil lived in the same college as strangers to each other." Here we have one of the most accomplished prose stylists of any age stumbling and staggering back and forth between two subjects, his tutor and himself, and dragging the reader along for the ride. The inadequately assigned gerund is not condemned in the grammar books among dangling modifiers because a gerund is a verbal noun, technically able to stand alone without modifying anything *(Skiing is cruising for a bruising.)* But in most instances the gerund is understood as having a subject, and when that subject is completely concealed from view by the use of the passive voice, confusion often results.

"By performing the initial examination with an endoscope adapted for taking biopsies, the patient is spared the trauma of repeated instrumentation." On first reading this sentence, we fear that this patient, too, has undertaken his own treatment, even to the point of performing endoscopy on himself. "On flexing the thigh sharply against the trunk, the patient experienced a recurrence of his pain." Did the patient flex his own thigh, or was it once again the invisible examiner?

"Without proposing regimentation or a restriction on innovations, the time has come for health professionals at all levels of training to survey objectively the devices they use." Here it is the editorialist who is not proposing regimentation or restriction, but that becomes clear only on a careful rereading of the sentence. It may be objected that the meaning of these examples can be determined by a moment's study, but that is hardly to the point. The reader of technical literature is not supposed to have to stop and figure things out word by word; there are crossword puzzles and murder mysteries for people who enjoy that sort of thing. Moreover, it is not always possible even on careful study to determine just what the writer means in a sentence like, "In explaining further his thinking on the amendment, the director was quoted by Evans as saying . . ." Who was doing the explaining here—the director (presumably the best interpreter of his own thinking) or Evans?

Nor are dangling modifiers the only culprits in midsentence thought shift. Here is a tortured muddle of a sentence in which an orphan relative clause is the problem: "He tripped while being pursued by a hornet, which caused a severe deltoid ligament tear." *Which* refers not to *hornet,* as we are first led to suppose, but to the act of tripping. The practice of letting an entire clause stand as the antecedent of the relative *which* is extremely common (15), and though not universally recognized as an error, it so often causes confusion that it should be avoided whenever possible.

In a review of a work on government intervention in medicine, we read that the author "has pulled no punches, some of them below the belt." Though the meaning may be obvious to all, a construction like this is offensively irregular. Comprehension depends on the reader's recognizing the two boxing metaphors here grotesquely intertwined, and not on literal interpretation of what has been written, which would be utterly impossible.

Though lack of coherence in sentence structure accounts for a very great number of faulty expressions, a wide variety of other stylistic irregularities contribute their share to the confusion. Consider the following hospital staff regulation: "Complete blood count and urinalysis are required on all patients undergoing general anesthesia. These tests must be completed within 48 hours of surgery." Yes, but before or after the surgery? It is of no use to point out that every physician reading the rule knows what it means; as a piece of legislation it simply does not stand up.

"Frequency of jaundice and seizures in patients receiving the drug was carefully monitored throughout the test period and for ninety days thereafter." The expression *frequency of jaundice* presumably means the incidence of jaundice as a function of the total number of patients. *Frequency of seizures,* however, surely implies a measurement of the rate of seizure activity in the individual. Regardless of how well designed and carefully executed the study may have been, the writer of the report has forfeited the credence and respect of his readers by lumping together two disparate ideas in a single word.

Other common sources of trouble are unintentional *doubles entendres* like *a tear in the lacrimal duct,* which is perfectly clear when spoken but causes at least momentary confusion when read. Words like *labial* and *cervical* are specific enough in a textbook of gynecology but may be equivocal in a more general context.

Much English prose, though containing no such ambiguities as

15. But only in English. Such a construction would not be tolerated in most other languages. Many allow a variation of the English phraseology in which a pronoun is inserted to distinguish this form of expression from a simple relative clause. Thus, in French this sentence would have to read, "He tripped while being pursued by a hornet, that which caused . . . etc."

these, is yet riddled with false starts and tangential trains of thought that distract and eventually exasperate the reader without his exactly knowing why. We gave examples of one kind of choppy, cluttered writing in Chapter 2 while discussing some of the peculiarities of the English adjective. Many of these impenetrably dense headline-style constructions result from misguided efforts at succinctness. Though *liver function studies* is surely preferable to *studies of the functions of the liver,* the products of this sort of compacting process are not uniformly successful; in *posttreatment traumatic functional impairment* a group of ideas have been crammed into fewer words than can possibly hold them. It is an ill-advised economy that conserves paper and ink at the expense of meaning itself.

Here is another instance of blatantly garbled language: "Select patients carefully (particularly the elderly) and follow them closely in line with the drug's precautions, warnings, contraindications and adverse reactions." The phrase in parentheses is syntactically adrift; *in line with* is a sloppy mode of expression, a mere formula, which with the preceding three words produces a ludicrous mixture of metaphors ("follow them closely in line"); but perhaps none of these faults is so gross as the bumbling reference to *the drug's precautions.*

In reading of a case of constrictive pericarditis we are surprised to learn that "Triamterene was prescribed to prevent potassium depletion," whereas we would have supposed that it was prescribed to promote diuresis. The grain of truth buried in this misstatement is that triamterene was chosen in preference to thiazide diuretics and others that increase excretion of potassium in order to avoid the potassium depletion that such drugs might have caused. The writer of the report has gotten into trouble by taking it for granted that the medical reader not only knows that triamterene is a diuretic but is familiar with its potassium-sparing property. Though his assumption may be generally valid, that does not change the fact that the sentence he wrote is false.

Most errors of this class probably would never get into print if the writer would only read over his work after an interval and edit passages that are not perfectly clear to one coming fresh to the material. Unfortunately many medical writers seem unwilling or unable to edit their own work, and too often the professional editor is more adept at rectifying purely grammatical irregularities than at detecting and amending more subtle but potentially more serious flaws in technical communication.

Medical editors and nonphysicians often express the criticism that medical writers make excessive use of the passive voice. The example of gobbledygook is not wholly to blame for this; in the following specimen it seems likely that the writer has been led astray chiefly by his quest for scientific detachment and objectivity: "Because of failure of response to conservative treatment, orthopedic consultation was sought." In this sentence, which has to do with the relationship among three persons, not one of those persons is mentioned. Instead, they are represented by nebulous concepts: the primary physician by *conservative treatment,* the specialist by *orthopedic consultation* and the patient—he for whose sake the science of medicine exists—by *failure of response.*

Notice how, in the following sentence, whenever the opportunity presents itself for the writer to make an honest, straightforward statement about people, he sidesteps it and serves up instead a hash of gerunds and passive constructions: "By initiating two new programs on a pilot project basis and by re-emphasizing the use of an ongoing program, it is hoped that the goal will be met of maintaining the same quality of health care while reducing the length of hospital stay."

Not the least objectionable features of this barbarous style of writing are its general air of awkwardness and untidiness and its potential for blurring or even burying the writer's meaning. "On auscultation a murmur was heard" and "At laparotomy the gallbladder was found to be acutely inflamed" are probably no more clumsy than the melodramatic "Palpation revealed a nodule" or the long-winded "Firm pressure was associated with a marked increase in discomfort." But all four of these expressions are open to the objection that they neither identify the persons whose actions and relations are being described, nor give a clear picture of those actions and relations.

Besides leading to a stilted and graceless style of writing, excessive use of the passive voice can easily result in grammatical faults, ranging from the inelegant ("An advantage of early endoscopy is that it enables biopsy") to the grotesque ("It is felt that this lesion should be kept an eye on").

bibliography

Except for purely historical facts, and matters of common knowledge (which, though sometimes wrong, are never questioned), all statements to which no reference is directly appended will be found corroborated in one or more of the following works.

History of the English Language

Bodmer F: THE LOOM OF LANGUAGE. New York, WW Norton, 1944
Chaurand J: HISTOIRE DE LA LANGUE FRANÇAISE. Paris, Presses Universitaires de France, 1972
Jespersen O: GROWTH AND STRUCTURE OF THE ENGLISH LANGUAGE, 9th ed. Riverside, NJ. The Free Press, MacMillan, 1968
Lounsberry J: HISTORY OF THE ENGLISH LANGUAGE. New York, Henry Holt, 1907
McKnight G: THE EVOLUTION OF THE ENGLISH LANGUAGE FROM CHAUCER TO THE TWENTIETH CENTURY. (Original title: MODERN ENGLISH IN THE MAKING.) New York, Dover, 1968

Medical Terminology

BLAKISTON'S GOULD MEDICAL DICTIONARY, 3rd ed. New York, McGraw-Hill, 1972
DORLAND'S ILLUSTRATED MEDICAL DICTIONARY, 25th ed. Philadelphia, Saunders, 1974
Gordon B: CURRENT MEDICAL INFORMATION AND TERMINOLOGY, 4th ed. Chicago, American Medical Association, 1971
INTERNATIONAL CLASSIFICATION OF DISEASES, Eighth Revision. Public Health Service Publication No. 1693, Washington, DC Government Printing Office, 1967
Jablonski S: ILLUSTRATED DICTIONARY OF EPONYMIC SYNDROMES AND DISEASES. Philadelphia, Saunders, 1969
STANDARD NOMENCLATURE OF DISEASES AND OPERATIONS, 5th ed. New York, McGraw-Hill, 1961
STEDMAN'S MEDICAL DICTIONARY, 22nd ed. Baltimore, Williams & Wilkins, 1972

Word Origins

Dauzat A: DICTIONNAIRE ÉTYMOLOGIQUE. Paris, Librairie Larousse, 1938
d'Hauterives R: DICTIONNAIRE DES RACINES DES LANGUES EUROPÉENNES. Paris, Librairie Larousse, 1948

THE OXFORD ENGLISH DICTIONARY. Oxford, Clarendon Press, 1933
Shipley J: DICTIONARY OF WORD ORIGINS. New York, Philosophical Library, 1945

English Usage

Farmer J, Henley W: SLANG AND ITS ANALOGUES (reprint). New York, Arno, 1970
Follett W: MODERN AMERICAN USAGE: A GUIDE. New York, Hill and Wang, 1966
Fowler H: A DICTIONARY OF MODERN ENGLISH USAGE. New York, Oxford University Press, 1944
Mencken HL: THE AMERICAN LANGUAGE, 4th ed. New York, Alfred A. Knopf, 1937
Strunk W, White EB: THE ELEMENTS OF STYLE. New York, Macmillan, 1959

indexes

Index of Words and Phrases

General Index